KATHY SMITH

FEED MUSCLE
shrink fat diet

6 Weeks to the Best Shape of Your Life

A Revolutionary
Diet From America's
Fitness Expert

Meredith Books® Des Moines, Iowa

Meredith Books
1716 Locust Street
Des Moines, Iowa 50309–3023
meredithbooks.com

Printed in the United States of America.

First Edition.
Library of Congress Control Number: 2007934806
ISBN: 978-0-696-23832-1

SEE YOUR DOCTOR FIRST

This diet and fitness book is designed to provide helpful information on the subjects addressed. This book is sold with
the understanding that the author and publisher are not rendering medical, health, or other personal services. The suggestions for specific exercise routines, foods, and lifestyle recommendations are not intended to replace medical advice
or treatment by your physician. All questions and concerns regarding your health, metabolism, weight, nutrition, and
physical activity should be directed to your physician, particularly if you have any health problems or medical problems
(including if you are pregnant or lactating). All reasonable attempts have been made to include the most recent and fac-
tual research and medical reports regarding exercise and nutrition. However, there is no guarantee that future research,
particularly human studies, will not change the information presented here. Further, the Internet addresses in this book
were accurate at the time of printing. Individual needs vary, and no nutrition or exercise program will meet everyone's
needs. Be sure to consult your physician prior to following any of the suggestions presented in this book and also before
changing your diet or exercise routine. You should rely on your physician's advice regarding whether the suggestions
presented in this book are appropriate for you, and you should rely on your physician to establish your weight goal. The
author and publisher disclaim all liability associated with the recommendations and guidelines set forth in this book.

All of the success stories and before/after photos in this book were from people who have transformed their bodies
through Kathy Smith's diet and exercise programs. Some of them were specifically featured in her latest infomercial
product, called Project: YOU!™, which is distributed by Beachbody.com of Product Partners, LLC. Project: YOU!™
features the same principles as the Feed Muscle, Shrink Fat program.

The brands listed are meant to give you an idea of the types of products being referred to. They are not endorsed by
the author or publisher, nor have the products or companies who produce the products endorsed the diet or fitness
plan in this book.

TABLE *of* CONTENTS

ACKNOWLEDGMENTS

For all those who helped make this book a reality. First, to my agent Bonnie Solow who challenged me with her wisdom, strength, passion, and soulful spirit to take my message to a new level.

Thank you to Kristin Loberg, my writer, who has extraordinary skills in capturing my voice, vision, and passion, as well as an unflappable attitude under pressure. Anybody who gets up and runs 10 miles or teaches a Spinning class before sitting down to write is clearly a kindred spirit.

To the redheaded dynamo Suzie Dimpfl, who excels at the art of describing how to do an exercise. Her unrivaled knowledge of the body's mechanics was key in completing this project.

Thank you to Amanda Stein, M.S., R.D., a well-rounded nutrition expert, for putting complex biological information into terms anyone can understand.

My friend Charna Nissenson was invaluable in creating the recipes. This book marks one more experience we've shared over the last 30 years. Her delectable cooking is exquisite and yet sensible to make.

To the entire team at Meredith Books: A special thanks goes out to Stephanie Karpinske, who helped shape and finetune the final manuscript. To Ken Carlson whose eye for design brought many pages to life. And to Lisa Berkowitz, who always made me feel that my book was in capable hands.

To Valorie Weaver and Dr. Jennifer Ashton for taking the time to write a foreword. Thanks, Dr. Ashton, for lending your perspective as a practicing physician and champion of healthy living.

To all the restaurants that contributed recipes. And thanks to Luiz Ratto for sharing recipes from his own book, *The Healthy Table*.

To the team at Beachbody.com and Product Partners, LLC, and especially to Carl Daikeler and all the Project: YOU!™ participants. You keep me inspired and your dedication is deeply appreciated.

Thanks to Matt "MattMan" McConkey for his support. It's not an easy task working with the Queen of Multitasking (that would be me). The system just wouldn't work without his holding it together.

To "Jackie-Girl" Mendes: You are such a light, energy, and master of crisis management. You have seen me through thick and thin. Thanks for your support, friendship, and also your gourmet taste. (Thanks to your mom too.)

And last but not least, thanks to Russ Kamalski for always believing in my vision to make the world a healthier place. And to my family—especially Katie and Perrie—for always bringing a smile to my face and keeping me grounded.

FOREWORD

We are beginning an exciting time in health, medicine, and wellness—characterized by disease prevention and good lifestyle habits. Yet ironically our struggle with weight and exercise has never been greater. One of every three Americans is obese, so the messages that we hear every single day are clearly just not getting through.

As a physician I see patients every day who have a variety of issues stemming from poor diet and fitness. Ranging from depression and low self-esteem to sleep apnea and high blood pressure, these problems span the spectrum from annoying to life-threatening. We know that being overweight and inactive increases our risk factors for heart disease, diabetes, and many types of cancer. But knowledge and action are often two totally distinct things. People just can't seem to get from point A to point C in their struggle with weight, nutrition, and fitness.

Why? Well, it's surely not due to lack of resources. There are countless books, magazines, videos, blogs, and, yes, doctors out there telling people what to do. What sets this book apart is that Kathy delves into the areas of science, nutrition, and exercise physiology and then finishes it all off with what may be the most important element of all: a healthy dose of reality. She understands that even the best intentions can run amok when the demands of everyday life set in—when work is crazy, the kids need attention, and fatigue and frustration are knocking at the door. But she also understands how to nudge us back on track. Her scientific but down-to-earth plan is made for anyone who wants to change for the better. And it doesn't take forever to do. Kathy's *Feed Muscle, Shrink Fat Diet* lives up to its title without relying on unhealthy gimmicks.

Kathy's three-part formula of feeding muscle, shrinking fat, and improving fitness addresses the very core of what is needed to achieve and maintain a healthy body. Her recipe does what I have always insisted is at the heart of a successful living plan. It focuses on "in versus out." Put simply: You have to burn more than you consume!

Kathy explains the different effects of the foods you choose to put "in" your body and then gives you her best tools to get the calories "out" (in the form of exercise). By taking very complex human physiology and breaking it down into simple, user-friendly principles, she makes it easy to understand how different foods affect the two main types of cells in your body: fat and muscle. The result? Eating deliciously but with a purpose. Everything on

Kathy's menu has a precise nutritional goal—nothing is wasted!

Americans are lucky. We have access to a very modern and often hedonistic style of living, but like any sword, this one has another edge. We do not like to deprive ourselves of any reward. We work hard and we like to play hard too! All of this play, however, often leaves us overweight and underfit. We need to break this cycle of unhealthy living before diabetes, hypertension, heart disease, and cancer take over. To win this battle we need all the help we can get. This is not a fight we can risk losing. Our lives and the lives of our children depend on our being healthy and thriving, not simply existing.

Sure, you may be tired of repeatedly trying and failing to become fit and trim. You are not alone. But remember, failure is NOT an option when the fight is for your life, wellness, and nutrition! Every body, physiologically and psychologically, has the potential for success. All you need to find is the right message delivered by the right messenger. This book contains that message, and there is no question that when it comes to diet and fitness Kathy is the right messenger.

Best wishes to a healthier you!

Jennifer Ashton, M.D.

Dr. Jennifer Ashton is a graduate of Columbia College, Columbia University, and Columbia College of Physicians and Surgeons in New York City. Currently Dr. Ashton practices general obstetrics and gynecology, specializing in adolescent gynecology at Women's Comprehensive Care. She is also a regular medical contributor on the Fox News Channel and featured guest on Fox Radio Live. She resides in Englewood, New Jersey, with her physician husband and their two children.

A LETTER FROM KATHY

Sometimes it is hard for me to believe I'm in my 50s because I enjoy life more than ever and I feel great. What is my secret to healthy living, boundless energy, and successful weight control? Muscle. In fact it is the backbone of my six-week *Feed Muscle, Shrink Fat Diet* program. Fueling your muscle cells through nutrition and exercise helps you achieve an ideal weight and optimum fitness level.

By the end of this book, you will have a new understanding of what I mean when I say "muscle." Muscle is more than the triceps, biceps, and abdominals that immediately come to mind. Muscle is about preventing disease. It is about coordination, balance, agility, and staying active. In short, muscle is about all those qualities we equate with youth such as endurance, energy, and relatively easy weight management.

I discovered this secret early in my life. My father died of a heart attack when I was just 17. At 19 I lost my mother in a plane crash. It was a depressing time for me, and that is when I started running and doing aerobics. It didn't take long for me to understand the value of the good feelings that came with being in shape. I started working on a second college degree, studying dance, kinesiology, exercise physiology, and nutrition. When I moved to Los Angeles, I became a certified fitness trainer and started creating my fitness programs, which eventually led me to develop my revolutionary Matrix plan—a total body approach to fitness. The Matrix system was a huge success, and my fitness books, DVDs, videos, and workout music CDs continue to be best sellers.

My new *Feed Muscle, Shrink Fat Diet* book combines all the secrets I have learned over the years with the latest science from the fitness and nutrition world to show you the way I eat and exercise to stay in the best shape of my life. The program is easy and adaptable, accessible no matter where you live, and fun.

My inspiration for this new diet really took off with the help of Amanda Stein M.S., R.D., a friend of mine who is also a registered dietitian. She is great at explaining basic concepts about diet and physiology. One of Amanda's mantras is to think of your body as only two things: muscle cells and fat cells. Everything you do feeds either one or the other. Granted this is an oversimplification of some complex biochemical pathways. But the underlying lesson is empowering: If you know how to feed and support your muscle cells, you stand a greater chance of shrinking your fat cells and shaping a tighter, leaner body.

My *Feed Muscle, Shrink Fat Diet* book turns this concept into a road map that you can apply to your everyday life *without* having to give up all your favorite foods. It takes all the guesswork out of losing weight and it will help you get into the best shape of your life.

It all comes down to this: Life is an endless series of choices. *This outfit or that one? Turn right or left? Now or later? Exercise before work or sleep in? Ice cream sundae or fresh fruit?* I want to help you automatically make good decisions that will ultimately allow you to participate in life at its fullest. With the Feed Muscle, Shrink Fat Diet, you will discover how even simple choices can improve your life. I know it is possible because thousands of you have shared your success stories and gratitude with me. I'm proud to have inspired the best in so many people. Let me assure you that you inspire me too.

Now let's get moving!

Kathy Smith

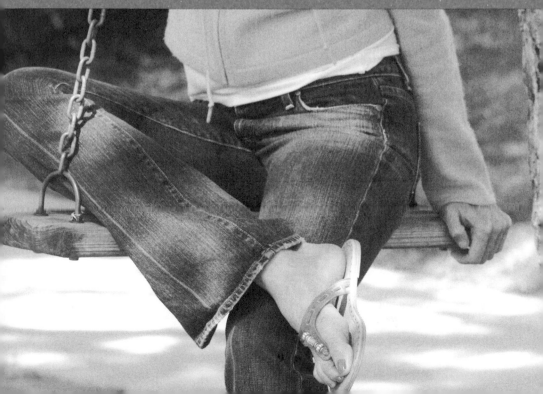

INTRODUCTION

Simply by picking up this book, you have taken an important step toward getting in the best shape of your life. It's an exciting (and delicious) adventure.

What would you say if I asked you what it means to be in the best shape of your life? Maybe it's losing 20 pounds and seeing real muscle definition in your arms, abs, and legs. Maybe it's lowering your cholesterol and risk for diabetes. Maybe it's feeling more energetic and accomplishing more throughout the day. And maybe it's all of these things plus more.

Chances are you have picked up this book because a voice inside your head is telling you that it is time to make a change. You want to take the weight off and adopt a healthier lifestyle, but you wonder how hard it will be. Making lifestyle changes, even little ones, can seem overwhelming at first. You ask: How can I avoid my usual habits? Will I feel deprived or hungry? Is this program doable given the time I have and the commitments I already have made?

My Feed Muscle, Shrink Fat Diet is the answer. It is a simple, straightforward strategy for taking the weight off and gaining health. It incorporates a variety of satisfying foods and it has the right balance of structure and adaptability to honor your personal preferences and power of choice.

You will finish my six-week Feed Muscle, Shrink Fat program with the knowledge and inspiration to stay on a healthy path for the rest of your life. The closer you stick to my program, the faster you will see results—and be in the best shape of your life.

THE BIG PAYOFFS

Whatever your reasons for changing how you eat and starting an exercise routine, I want you to keep one thing in mind: Being in shape has much greater rewards than a smaller waistline or a lower resting heart rate. Thousands of people who use my programs and work out with me tell me the biggest payoff is how different they *feel*. Weight loss might be first and foremost in your mind, but the benefits of the Feed Muscle, Shrink Fat program don't end there. In every area of your life, you will notice results that include:

- greater confidence and self-esteem
- a new clarity on life that helps trump daily stress
- better sleep and more energy day after day
- a medical transformation in terms of lower blood pressure, lower cholesterol level, and improved bone health
- diabetes prevention or control
- reduction in joint pain
- a stronger immune system
- a more youthful appearance

- a feeling of more control of your life and future
- ability to navigate more easily through stressful times
- feeling more accomplished both at work and home

In short, you will be a healthier, happier person. And you will be motivated to stick with my program because you'll feel a surge in your energy level. Remember, success tends to breed success, and this is especially true in maintaining a healthy body. When your life becomes richer, fuller, and more energized as a result of your efforts, you won't want to revert to your old, unhealthy lifestyle.

THE FEED MUSCLE, SHRINK FAT SCIENCE

When you walk by a magazine stand or bookstore, the numbers on the covers alone can cause confusion: "99 ways to drop 10," "86 ways to eat better," "25 secret fat-burning foods." The Feed Muscle, Shrink Fat program cuts through all the hype and focuses on the science behind food and our bodies.

The Feed Muscle, Shrink Fat program uses what scientists know about nutrition and exercise to make our bodies as efficient as possible 24/7. Small changes can mean the difference between burning fat during a workout (which is great) and breaking down muscle (which is not so great). My program focuses on:

- *what* you eat
- *when* you eat
- *how* and *how frequently* you exercise
- how you *combine* exercise with the proper food fuel

The Magic Feed Muscle, Shrink Fat Formula

Although the science behind my diet is complex, you have to remember only one simple equation:

$$Protein + Vitamin\ C + Fiber = Weight\ Loss$$

These are the ingredients your body craves for optimum health, and they are the backbone of every meal you eat on my program. I will teach you how to choose superfoods that fit this equation and that fuel muscles, shrink fat, and boost your overall health. Once you can identify the foods that contain these essential ingredients, knowing what to eat becomes second nature.

OVERVIEW OF THE SIX-WEEK DIET

My six-week Feed Muscle, Shrink Fat program puts you on the road to better health and fitness by combining diet with exercise and lifestyle changes. Let's take a quick tour of what you can expect to eat in the upcoming weeks.

Week 1: Fast Track 1 Breaks Your Bad Habits

Fast Track 1 helps you say goodbye to old habits and retrain your body with healthy, new ones. You'll make incremental improvements in how you eat that build one day at a time. In the first seven days of the Feed Muscle, Shrink Fat program, you follow a strict, daily structured food plan. But don't panic. There are good reasons for this. Fast Track 1 is the best way to jumpstart your weight loss and lay a solid foundation for the future.

The truth is that when you start a weight loss program, you are frustrated with how you look and what you have eaten. You feel out of control. That's OK. You're human. But to regain control you need to break that cycle of making unhealthy choices. This means following a rigid plan that doesn't require you to make too many decisions. Fast Track 1 rescues you from your old patterns and gives you clarity, focus, and motivation. Although there are restrictions the payoff is so great you will be thankful you made the commitment.

Fast Track 1 revs up your metabolism, extinguishes cravings, helps you establish discipline, and allows you to shed initial weight quickly. Some people lose 2 pounds during this first week, while others drop as much as 8 pounds! Some of that weight will be fat and some of it will be water. No matter how much you lose in just this first week, you will feel revitalized. You gain energy and inspiration. You start to feel more alive and alert. Your body begins to make shifts necessary to keep your metabolism running on high. Most important you can manage hunger and control portions without much thought.

Week 2: Fast Track 2 Puts Your Body in Balance

Starting on Day 8 your meal options expand. You start to reintroduce starchier carbohydrates into your diet while still continuing to lose weight and build lifelong healthy habits. You learn how to incorporate the right combination of nutrients into your diet so they work for you, not against you. This is when you start to really understand the weight loss formula that makes up the backbone of every meal: protein + vitamin C + fiber.

As in the first week, I give you an eating plan that consists of three balanced meals plus two snacks each day. There is no need to count calories or read nutrition labels because I've done all of the math for you. These meals are packed with nutrition and include some of the most delectable foods on the planet.

This week you also have the flexibility to substitute any of the meals in "Kathy's California Restaurant Favorites" (page 240), which features recipes from eateries near my Santa Monica hometown.

Weeks 3–6: Maximum Fat Burn Revs Up Your Weight Loss

By the time you reach Week 3, you have confidence in knowing what to eat, how much, and when. During the Maximum Fat Burn weeks, you learn to design your own healthy, nutritious meals that reflect more of your own needs, tastes, and personality. My goal is for you to learn how to be a creative chef who can stir up magic in the kitchen without much effort or thought. But again, don't worry. I give you fail-safe methods so that you don't have to guess at the right food choices.

THE FEED MUSCLE, SHRINK FAT RECIPES

I love to eat and I believe the ritual of creating meals and sharing those meals with loved ones is important. So I refuse to eat bland, boring food. Many people think that "healthy" equates with unsatisfying and flavorless. Wrong! You will be excited by the luscious, full-flavor foods you can eat on this plan and still lose weight. I have created more than 100 delicious recipes that will make you forget you are on a "diet."

None of these meals requires extensive planning, expensive grocery shopping, or access to specialty food stores. I include quick, on-the-go ideas and recipes that you can try when you have more time. No matter where you live, you'll be able to follow this plan. More than anything this program is about flavor, nutrition, variety, and convenience!

YOUR 10-MINUTE MATRIX WORKOUT

Exercise is a critical piece of the Feed Muscle, Shrink Fat program, but there is no need to spend hours in the gym. My exercise routines are based on my Matrix workout, which is one of the most *efficient* ways to exercise. In fact it is so efficient that you start with quick 10-minute daily workouts during Week 1 and Week 2. During the following weeks you add more time and more intensity for maximum calorie-burning.

Ten minutes may not seem like enough, but trust me, you experience high-quality training. This breakthrough approach to exercise uses the body's own weight as resistance to condition every square inch, improve coordination, balance, and flexibility, and strengthen your cardiovascular system. With this workout you will bend, twist, lunge, reach, and lift. In other words you strengthen the same muscles that you use in everyday life, lifting grocery bags or cleaning your house. This holistic style of training ultimately protects you against the aches, pains, and risk of injury that accompany age. It works on a wide variety of body types, and in six weeks you will discover a whole new you.

Starting in Week 2, you combine my Matrix exercises with cardio workouts and burst training to redefine your waistline, sculpt arms and legs, lift your butt, tighten your thighs, and more. All the details of this revolutionary system are provided in Part 2 (page 83). You also will have options to add additional resistance to the Matrix workout with dumbbells and to incorporate a walking program.

THE LAWS TO LIVING LEAN

In the real world losing weight and getting in shape take more than just learning about nutrition and exercise. There are a multitude of lifestyle habits that can affect how many calories you burn in a day. So you must also learn to deal with everyday issues that can prevent you from maintaining a healthy lifestyle. I share my Laws to Living Lean, which are my own secrets to a healthy lifestyle. These Laws are in Part 3 (page 146) and cover:
- coping with stress
- managing cravings for sweets
- getting enough sleep
- making healthy choices in restaurants
- dealing with mental and physical plateaus
- learning how to tune in to your own connection between mood and food—and mood and motivation

As a busy mom and business owner, I know that life can get in the way of staying at the top of my game. With my techniques for keeping motivated and taking good care of yourself, you can stay at the top of your game too.

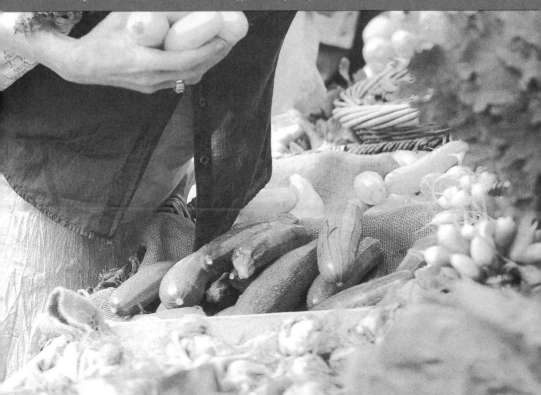

PART 1: THE DIET

In just six weeks you will learn to eat based on my scientific weight loss formula and to exercise effectively in just 10 minutes a day.

Welcome to the training grounds where you teach your body little by little to lose weight and remain fit and lean for the long term. I want you to know from the start that the Feed Muscle, Shrink Fat program isn't an all-or-nothing approach. You learn a way of living that you can sustain for the long term because you can customize it to fit your lifestyle, your food preferences, and your needs. All I ask is that you make the most of these next six weeks and tune in to how your body is changing and feeling. You reboot and recalibrate your body one day and one meal at a time. You start to see results immediately, and even more accumulate over time.

You may think you are changing your body from the outside, given the foods you eat and workouts you do, but more than you can probably imagine is going on inside at a cellular level. You positively affect and modify your metabolism, your motor skills and neurons, your muscle tissue, your digestive system, your skeletal system, your heart and lung capacity, and so much more. And these significant transformations take time.

So take a deep breath, relax, and get ready to discover a whole new you. If you have not eaten well in a while, be patient with yourself as you begin to make these important shifts. Like the old adage goes, life is what you make of it. Simply choose to be the best that you can be, and positive changes will occur in your life in ways you never dreamed possible.

Success Story: Amy Copeland

"I hit 220 pounds after the birth of my son. A year later I began using Kathy Smith's step video daily. I changed my eating habits and learned to eat the right foods. I lost 40 pounds, and I was hooked! I became a regular on Kathy's Internet message boards. Kathy answered many of my questions and encouraged me on my journey. I have lost a total of 71 pounds and am now at my goal weight. I would not have been able to do it without Kathy's help. Thank you, Kathy, for being such an inspiration."

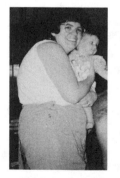
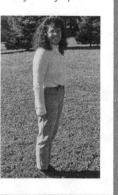

BEFORE YOU START

You need to become mentally and physically prepared to embark on this exciting journey. So here are some things to consider before you start.

END BODY CHAOS AND YO-YO DIETING

By the time people come to me, they have often tried many different diet and fitness programs, and nothing has given them long-term results. They lose weight initially and then regain all of it—and sometimes even more. They then try something else and the cycle repeats, creating weight fluctuation that results in what I call body chaos.

A yo-yo dieting cycle of weight loss and weight gain is not only mentally defeating, but it also generates chaos that puts the body on the defensive and metabolism on hold. You store energy as fat and use muscle for fuel. That is exactly the opposite of what you want to do. To make things worse each attempted "quick fix" pushes your metabolism further into chaos, making it increasingly hard to lose weight and keep it off for good.

Imagine the toll this takes on your body when the pendulum swings back and forth on your metabolism. One day your body works in starvation mode; the next it packs away excess energy as fat because you ate more than your body needed. This cycle ultimately sacrifices health and the ability to maintain a steady metabolism.

Body chaos goes much deeper than just metabolism. When I see people struggling with body chaos, I immediately wonder what else is happening when they deprive their bodies of the nutrition and exercise they need. I think about clogged arteries, thinning bones, an overworked heart, and fat deposits around organs. The No. 1 killer is still heart disease, even among women. And while one in eight women will have breast cancer, one in *two* women over age 50 will have a fracture from osteoporosis.

It is natural to focus on outer fitness when we look in the mirror every day. But keep in mind that outer beauty starts with inner health, which is what the Feed Muscle, Shrink Fat program helps you achieve.

IDENTIFY WHAT TYPE OF EATER YOU ARE

Identifying what kind of an eater you are is valuable at the start of a program. From working with dietitians and doctors over the years, I know that recognizing your usual eating habits and behaviors from the get-go makes the process of shifting your lifestyle easier. It can pinpoint where you need to focus your efforts during the upcoming weeks on this program. I won't ask you to completely change your eating behavior; I prefer the word *shift*. It is human nature to resist change, but making slight shifts for the better is a much more inviting proposition. I simply want you to begin to make small adjustments to what you already do, which can start with understanding your relationship with food. There are typically four types of eating behavior. Which type describes you best? (It is common to see yourself in more than one of these definitions.)

Kathy's Secret: I recommend that you see your doctor to share your weight loss goals prior to beginning my program. Make this a team effort. Your doctor also can help you address any special medical needs or issues unique to you, as well as determine an ideal weight goal that will guide you as you follow the diet.

Emotional eater. Is it a need for comfort that starts you eating? Stress? Anxiety? Around 60 to 70 percent of people have an emotional attachment to food. There is a clear biological reason for that: When you were a baby, you got your nourishment from Mom's breast or a bottle. It was also your way of receiving love, so food became associated with positive emotions. The trick now is to know whether you eat for nourishment and fuel or just for that feel-good sensation that often accompanies eating. For the emotional eater keeping a journal will be an important way to track feelings and begin to see patterns in eating behaviors. (See "Start a Diary," page 21.) The journal will help you identify better ways of dealing with emotions, ways that don't entail overeating. (See "Detach Mood from Food," page 154, for more tips about breaking unhealthy habits and finding satisfying substitutions.)

Volume eater. This type of eater is often an emotional eater too, although not always. Many people fill themselves with food to avoid uncomfortable feelings such as exhaustion, pain, and stress. Downing an entire bag of potato chips when you are under stress is a classic example. For others volume eating is just their style of eating. They prefer to eat large portions spaced far apart with little or no snacking in between. This kind of eating is not necessarily tied to emotions. Volume eaters will find lots of options in the Feed Muscle, Shrink Fat Diet that allow for large portions, particularly in the vegetable category.

Grazer. If you are a multitasker who tends to be time-conscious and deadline-driven, you might be a grazer who grabs food whenever you can. Grazers skip large meals, preferring to eat mini meals every two to three hours. Grazers will love my Feed Muscle, Shrink Fat program because it recommends eating every three to four hours to keep metabolism humming and blood sugar balanced.

Off-balance eater. When you work 10 or more hours a day and don't have much control over your meals, it is easy to become an off-balance eater. You may avoid eating during the day and then arrive home on empty—physically and emotionally. At that point the house gets eaten. For the off-balance eater, it is either feast or famine. The off-balance eater will benefit tremendously from journaling. (See "Start a Diary," page 21.) It will help you zero in on what is happening in your life to sabotage weight loss goals. On the Feed Muscle, Shrink Fat plan, you learn how to stock your kitchen so when you have an off-balance day, you are prepared to feast on a nutritious meal.

You can achieve nutritional success no matter what kind of eater you are, but being aware of your habits can help you reach your goals faster and maintain them for the rest of your life. If you are not sure at the start of this program what type of eater describes you best, keeping a journal will answer that question.

Kathy's Secret: It's important to identify your problem foods. Think for a moment: What foods can't you eat in moderation, no matter what? Keep in mind that even so-called healthy foods can impede weight loss when eaten in massive quantities. When you crave these foods, it is hard to say no. When cravings strike try popping a piece of gum or a breath freshener strip in your mouth. Or head outside for a 10-minute walk, which is enough to increase your circulation and improve your mood naturally. The mere act of changing your environment can cut the craving.

MAKE "CONSISTENCY" YOUR MANTRA

When people ask me for the secret to health and fitness, I advise: Be consistent, be consistent, be consistent. Self-care should not be an on-and-off proposition. Unfortunately people fall into the trap of repeatedly neglecting themselves. If they don't have time to do a regular workout, they abandon the whole thing and lose momentum for days or weeks. If they see food only in terms of good or bad, they fall into long cycles of overindulging and undernourishing.

I eat and exercise in a way that serves me, my health, and my body, without ever going to extremes. This is the kind of consistency I'm talking about, and it is what I will help you achieve for yourself. Finding your own unique version of consistency will be key to your success. Ideally you will figure out within the menu plans and recipes what works for you. Then you can adapt this program to your life and maintain it on a consistent basis.

How do you find consistency? By having motivators. Motivators can be anything—an upcoming trip to Hawaii, the desire to run a 10K, or even a medical scare in the family that made you think about your own health.

Kathy's Secret: Shoot for progress—not perfection. Instead of scolding yourself for overeating, as you may have done in the past, imagine talking to yourself the way you'd talk to a friend—with encouragement and humor! So instead of focusing on the thought "I wasn't perfect today," how about "I did the best I could; I had a hectic day!" By giving yourself a powerful affirmation and using more positive self-talk, you can start to tame the wild beast of perfectionism.

Whenever people start a weight loss program, I ask them to write down all the reasons they want to lose weight. It is likely that they begin with simple reasons like "I want thinner thighs." But when pushed they add other reasons like "I want more energy," "I want better sleep," "I want to spend more quality time with my kids," "I want to live longer," or "I want a better sex life." I encourage you to look at the big picture. This nutrition and exercise program affects much more than your weight; it affects your entire life.

When you're feeling low your motivators will remind you why you have decided to make these changes. Have faith in your power to change.

THINK MUSCLE, NOT FAT

It is far too easy to direct your thoughts to the negative when trying to lose weight. Your mind can focus on belly rolls and trouble spots, filling you with feelings of frustration. Is there any way to put a positive spin on that? Yes! Stop worrying about fat and start thinking about *muscle*. Muscle is at the core of the Feed Muscle, Shrink Fat program. But "feeding muscle" is not about building bulky arms and legs. It's about power, energy, balance, coordination, speedy recovery from illness and injury, and quick mental and physical response time. Above all it is about keeping your body young.

Just that one slight shift in your mindset—from the negative to the exceptionally positive—can automatically help you make smarter, healthier decisions. I will show you exactly how you can "think yourself thin" and employ the power of positive thinking to effect the changes you want to see in your body.

GET ONLINE SUPPORT

You will find valuable support and more tools to help you in your weight loss and fitness goals at my website, kathysmith.com. If you register you will have access to a variety of resources, including new recipes and grocery lists. You also can join us in virtual workout rooms.

CALCULATE YOUR BMI

To figure out the percent of fat to lean muscle mass in your body, calculate your body mass index (BMI). BMI is a measure of weight relative to height. Ideal weight and fat to lean ratios vary by sex, age, and height. The average adult male should be 15 to 18 percent; the average adult female should be 22 to 25 percent. To calculate your BMI and view charts that indicate ideal weight ranges, use the online calculator at my website, kathysmith.com. Plug in your height and weight to find out your BMI with just the click of a mouse.

START A DIARY

Keeping a journal can maximize your fitness and nutrition results on this program. You can download a Total Control Nutrition & Exercise Diary template at kathysmith.com, or create your own journal using any notebook. Divide your journal into sections that cover the following:

Foods. Keep track of what you eat every day.

Workouts. Enter what workouts you do. Be sure to include all physical activities because they all have an impact on your fitness level and weight loss. For example, record that you took the stairs rather than the elevator or that you walked instead of drove to the store.

Hunger levels. Record your hunger levels before and after meals. Use a scale of 1 to 5, where 1 means "stuffed" and 5 means "starving." A 3 is "normal," and that is where you want to be most of the time.

Weekly goals. Set as many goals as you like, but be realistic.

Emotions. Record what is happening in your life too. Write down your thoughts, what mood you are in, what life events are most affecting you, and so on. Were you happy and lighthearted or edgy and annoyed? Your mental attitude has a lot to do with your physical energy, and you can learn to use happiness as a motivator in your success.

If you feel "ruined" by a day of overeating and little or no exercise, it is especially important to record your thoughts and the happenings of the day. There could be days when you are on the go and do not pack a meal. So you go to a fast-food joint. When you feel tired and overworked, you may fall prey to comfort foods that are high in fat and calories. Be sure to make the entry, even if you would rather skip it or pretend the day did not exist. Seeing these difficult days charted on paper will help you identify behavioral patterns, pitfalls, and roadblocks that prevent you from being a successful eater. It can help explain why and when you eat certain foods. And this in turn will help you make positive changes.

Everyone has days of minor derailments. Remind yourself that tomorrow is another day. It is not the end of the world. Be diligent with your entries, and at the end of six weeks you will have a chronicle of your progress to reflect upon with pride and satisfaction.

STOCK YOUR KITCHEN

It may shock you to know that half of all Americans eat out every day. More than 25 percent of what we eat comes from restaurants. As a result Americans consume between 400 and 500 more calories per day than they did just 20 years ago. The truth is that when we are not at home, it is easy to overeat with unhealthy foods that wind up in our fat cells. Your chance of weight loss success rises dramatically if you commit to planning your meals. If you always have healthy options in the house, you are less likely to eat whatever is available and regret it later. Your first step is to stock your kitchen with the right staples.

When you start the Feed Muscle, Shrink Fat program, shopping for food can be intimidating. That bright supermarket suddenly becomes a place full of forbidden goodies and unhealthy choices. But do not be nervous. The first step to enjoyable and effective shopping is done at home: Simply decide what you need before you go to the store.

Prior to starting Week 1: Fast Track 1, make a list of items you need from the grocery store based on which meals you choose. You will find the first week of meals—breakfasts, lunches, and dinners—on page 45; the accompanying recipes start on page 164. While I indicate specific meals on Day 1, Day 2, Day 3, and so

KITCHEN STAPLES

Stock up on these items that should be on hand at all times. On the Feed Muscle, Shrink Fat plan, you will use some of them every single day.

Olive and canola oils
Canola or olive oil cooking spray
Balsamic and rice wine vinegars
Egg whites. For ease try Eggology egg whites from the refrigerated section.
Fat-free or light cow's milk or soymilk
Low-fat cottage cheese
Low-fat cheeses and yogurts
Grated Parmesan cheese
Protein powder, such as whey, soy, or egg white
Fresh vegetables, such as broccoli, asparagus, spinach, cauliflower, jicama, celery, mushrooms, tomatoes, cucumbers, and sweet peppers
Fresh fruit, such as apples, pears, and berries
Salsa
Dijon mustard
Light mayonnaise, such as those made with soy or canola oil
Lettuce, such as iceberg, baby greens, romaine, arugula, endive, and kale
Fresh herbs, such as parsley, cilantro, basil, chives, oregano, thyme, and rosemary
Spices, such as cinnamon, chili powder, lemon pepper, curry, and cayenne pepper
Lemons
Garlic and fresh ginger
Unsalted raw nuts
Lean deli meat slices, such as turkey or chicken
Turkey bacon and/or turkey sausage
Water-packed tuna. "Light" tuna has less mercury than "white" or albacore.
Fresh fish
Flaxseed oil or meal
Natural nut butters. Almond has less saturated fat than peanut.
Whole grain cereal. Choose those with more than 8 grams of fiber per serving.
Steel-cut oatmeal, such as old-fashioned or McCann's Quick & Easy Irish Oatmeal
Multigrain and whole grain pastas. Try Barilla Plus® and Ronzoni Healthy Harvest®.
Whole grain breads and tortillas. Try Ezekiel® breads and Mission Low-Carb® tortillas.
Whole grain brown rice. In a hurry? Look for Rice Expressions® in the freezer section.

on, feel free to substitute meals from other days. For example, if on Day 3 you do not want red snapper for dinner, try salmon or orange roughy. I want this plan to be flexible and meet your needs, so choose the foods that interest you. If I suggest something that you cannot tolerate, simply choose something else.

The only rule is that you should not choose a meal from Week 2: Fast Track 2 during Week 1: Fast Track 1. Also I recommend that you plan your meals just a few days at a time. This will encourage you to buy fresh foods that you will use before they spoil.

YOU ARE READY TO START!

One final tip I would like to share: Focus on waist size, not pounds. Don't worry about what the scale reads. As you trim body fat and increase lean muscle mass, you might not see a huge difference on the scale right away. So instead of using the scale to gauge your progress, measure your waistline once a week and track the results. Chances are you will see your measurements become smaller!

Success Story: Carol Conforti

"At first the diet was a little tough because I was used to eating more. But then I realized I was losing a pound a day and suddenly it felt easy! With Kathy's program you'll get better results, and you'll never get bored. I went from 146 pounds to 135 in two weeks and shed an entire dress size. I couldn't believe how quickly it happened!"

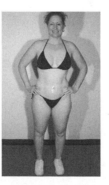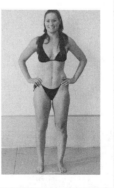

Photos provided by Beachbody.com

THE SCIENCE BEHIND THE PROGRAM

The basic premise of the Feed Muscle, Shrink Fat Diet is exactly as its name implies: If you learn how to "feed" your muscle cells, you can shrink your fat cells. To understand how this works, think of the body as being made up of these three things:

- muscle cells
- fat cells
- water

When you eat nutrient-dense foods, you feed muscle cells. (Nutrient-dense foods, such as kiwi and broccoli, have lots of vitamins and minerals but few calories.) By feeding your muscles you are not actually creating more muscle but rather making your existing muscles stronger. The result is that you gain critical muscle mass. The benefits of feeding muscles are clear: more energy, reduced food cravings, feelings of fullness, and an improved sense of well-being.

By contrast when you eat calorie-dense foods like those filled with sugar, salt, and fat, you feed your fat cells, which then expand and get bigger. (Calorie-dense foods, such as macaroni and cheese, have lots of calories but few vitamins and minerals.)

While it is true that once you have a fat cell, you can't get rid of it, the good news is getting fat has little to do with how many fat cells you have. It has more to do with how big those fat cells are. Fat cells can only duplicate at two points in our lives: when we are babies and during puberty. Once our fat cells mature in our teenage years, we essentially have those fat cells the rest of our lives. So fat cells can neither be created nor destroyed—but they can be *shrunk*.

This is an oversimplification of the body's complex anatomy and physiology. But it helps explain the importance of why you must "feed" your muscles—and not your fat—if you want to lose weight.

FAT FACT

A 100-pound person and a 300-pound person can have the same number of fat cells. But the 300-pound person is likely consuming too many calorie-dense foods that feed the fat cells, causing them to get bigger—and therefore heavier—than they are in the 100-pound person.

WHAT IS MUSCLE?

It is important to understand what makes muscle so magical. As we age retaining lean tissue—or muscle—is perhaps the greatest secret to looking youthful and feeling our best. Yet people forget how powerful muscle is to overall health.

Take a minute to consider some of the body parts that rely on our ability to move muscles, whether voluntary or involuntary. Muscle action pumps lymph through lymphatic vessels as part of our immune system. Breathing provides oxygen to the cells and depends on muscles. Muscles move food down through the digestive tract where nutrients are absorbed. Muscle activity in the skin allows us to perspire and maintain our temperature. And let us not forget the most important muscle of all: the heart. It is the primary means by which we stay alive as it continuously delivers oxygen and nutrients to cells. If we view the muscular system as an organ upon which other systems rely, we can then understand why it is so important to keep it well nourished and maintained.

Strengthening your muscles helps your bones too. The muscles you engage when you lift a weight put pressure on your bones, essentially forcing them to get stronger and stave off the brittle-bone disease, osteoporosis. That is important because a recent study found that loss of bone density may be an even better predictor of death from atherosclerosis (hardening of the arteries) than cholesterol levels.

Because muscle is in constant use by your body just to keep it alive and functioning, it is easy to understand how it also can affect weight, metabolism, and the ability to burn fat. In fact muscle is a *high-maintenance* tissue. That means it requires a lot of energy in the form of calories to keep it in good working order.

Even when a muscle appears to be at rest, a certain amount of sustained contraction is going on in its tiny fibers. This is called muscle tone, and it is a response to nerve impulses originating in the spinal cord. Muscle tone is what allows us to maintain posture and hold our heads up.

What does all this mean for weight loss? Simply put the more lean muscle you have, the faster your metabolism will be. High metabolism boosts your body's constant burning of calories, which ultimately leads to fat loss. Your muscles will burn calories whether you swim laps or just sit on the couch watching television.

The amount of lean muscle mass you carry relative to the rest of your body weight is a huge factor in whether your metabolism is moving along at 25 mph or zooming up to 500 mph.

WHAT IS FAT?

In contrast with muscle, fat is relatively inactive. It does not burn a lot of calories and, as you may have experienced, it seems to build up quickly and go away slowly. But fat does have a function. No one can have a fat-free body and be healthy at the same time. We need fat for insulation, protection, energy, and even to think. In fact about two-thirds of the brain is composed of fat, and the protective sheath that covers communicating neurons is 70 percent fat.

But not all fats are equal. While they may all deliver the same calories (about 9 calories per gram), some provide important nutrients, while others can actually damage your health.

Essential Fatty Acids

When you digest the fat in food, it is broken down into fatty acid molecules that your body needs to function properly. Essential fatty acids are otherwise known as the family of omega-3 and omega-6 fats that come from foods like fish, avocado, almonds, walnuts, flaxseeds, and olives. They are *essential* because the body cannot manufacture them. This is why it is so important that we get essential fatty acids from foods on a daily basis. The reason salmon is labeled as "brain food" is because it contains high-quality fat that is important for brain health. In fact all omega-3 fat has numerous health benefits. Researchers suspect that omega-3 fat found in fish also may protect against heart disease.

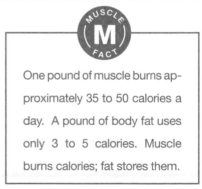

One pound of muscle burns approximately 35 to 50 calories a day. A pound of body fat uses only 3 to 5 calories. Muscle burns calories; fat stores them.

Dietary Fats

There are three kinds of dietary fat: saturated, unsaturated, and trans. When we eat these fats, we feed fat cells that can become extra padding on hips, thighs, the upper back, and backs of arms—especially when we consume high quantities of unhealthy fats. However, while most people could benefit from a cut in their dietary fat intake, it is unhealthy to completely eliminate it. Healthy fat helps fat-soluble vitamins like A, D, E, and K get around the body, creates sex hormones, lowers LDL (bad) cholesterol while elevating HDL (good) cholesterol, and contributes to the health of skin, eyes, nails, and hair. What's more, you need fat to burn fat. It also increases the satiety value of a meal, keeping you satisfied and feeling full.

There are not many foods I would label as "bad" because I think there is always a way to accommodate a food. But trans fats are bad, and I recommend that you remove them from your diet entirely. Trans fats are synthetic fats found in foods like french fries, margarine, potato chips, and anything else with partially hydrogenated oil. Trans fats can be threatening to your health, regardless of your level of fitness. They increase levels of LDL (bad) cholesterol and decrease levels of HDL (good) cholesterol. They have been shown to disrupt communication between cells in your brain. Nutrition labels must now list trans fat content. Another way to spot this fat is to look for "partially hydrogenated vegetable oil" on food labels.

Fat's Problem Areas

The body fat we should be especially vigilant about is the belly fat that lies deep inside. Doctors call this visceral fat because it wraps around your viscera—your vital organs such as your heart, liver, and lungs. Excess body fat generates hormones that can actually cause weight *gain* while preventing the production of healthy substances that can lead to weight *loss*. Recent studies in nutrition and medicine are currently changing the way doctors view obesity as they learn more about visceral fat and how it can change the body's internal chemistry. What this fat ultimately does is cause us to age more quickly and become vulnerable to disease. It has been linked to health problems including heart disease, type 2 diabetes, and metabolic syndrome, which is a cluster of risk factors that increases the chance of developing these diseases.

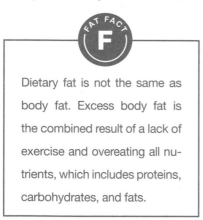

FAT FACT

Dietary fat is not the same as body fat. Excess body fat is the combined result of a lack of exercise and overeating all nutrients, which includes proteins, carbohydrates, and fats.

It is also important to note that visceral fat is not just a problem for overweight or obese people. Thin people also can have visceral fat if they are not fit. Abdominal fat is usually visible on most people, but visceral fat can be deep inside an outwardly "thin" person. The same holds true for fat that can line arteries and veins. We may not see this type of fat on the outside, but it can restrict blood flow and weaken the cardiovascular system. The good news is that you can burn fat through diet and exercise. And that is exactly what we are going to do.

Doing the Math: How Your Body Burns Fat

To lose one pound of fat you have to burn 3,500 more calories than you consume. For example, if you burned 500 more calories per day than you ate, in seven days you would have burned enough extra fat to lose one pound. For best results that 500-calorie daily deficit should be split between exercise and food. Burn about 250 calories more during your workout and eat about 250 calories less than you usually do.

The math is simple, but the human body is anything but! The equation works when you stick to moderate exercise and moderate food decreases. But many people want quick results, so they either restrict calories to starvation levels or exercise at extreme levels. Both wreak havoc on metabolism. Bodies are amazing machines. If food becomes scarce, bodies conserve every calorie. Similarly when you exercise frequently for long bouts, like several times a day, your metabolism will slow during the downtimes and will become more efficient during exercise. Your goal of burning more calories from exercise will be sabotaged by your body's attempt to survive. With my Feed Muscle, Shrink Fat program, you will find the right balance to burn fat and build lean muscle. No extremes. No deprivation.

WATER'S ROLE

Water makes up 68 to 72 percent of our blood. Being fully hydrated is one of the most basic secrets to weight loss. It helps your metabolism function properly and transports molecules, including the fat we are trying to burn. If you want to burn fat, it must be able to travel out of the body. Water provides that vehicle.

If the water in your blood drops below normal levels, muscle cells will give up water to support the flow necessary in the blood. When this happens dehydration occurs. The first sign of dehydration is actually hunger, so if you turn to food, you may sabotage weight loss goals.

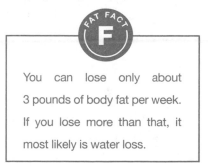

FAT FACT

You can lose only about 3 pounds of body fat per week. If you lose more than that, it most likely is water loss.

Do not worry about some water retention as your body begins to change as a result of the Feed Muscle, Shrink Fat program. The scale may be deceptive, showing water weight while you have actually lost fat weight. Also you will gain lean muscle mass, which like water is much heavier than fat. Fat is puffy and fluffy; water and muscle—two key elements to weight loss and superior fitness in general—are dense and heavy. You want as much water as possible available to keep your metabolism in high gear; it also will keep your endurance primed for extended workouts.

Low-Carb Diets

Diets that severely restrict carbohydrates may give people the illusion of sudden weight loss, and here is why. Cutting off carbohydrates forces the body to find other sources of energy. It likely turns to glycogen, which is simply stored carbohydrates in your muscles and liver. Once glycogen stores are tapped, water is released. (When a gram of glycogen is released in the body for fuel, 3 to 4 grams of water go with it.)

Some of the initial weight loss on the Feed Muscle, Shrink Fat plan can be attributed to water loss. That is OK. Eventually you will lose real weight in terms of real fat. It is important to realize that water levels in the body may fluctuate as you change your eating habits and increase your activity level. Not only do fat cells need water to convert fat to usable forms of energy, but your muscles also need water to perform. When you increase your physical activity, your muscles will store more glycogen with water to meet the demands you place on them. Likewise your bloodstream will carry more water, increasing the amount of blood traveling through your system to deliver much-needed oxygen to muscles. All of this action means a higher capacity to burn calories and shrink fat.

THE FEED MUSCLE, SHRINK FAT FORMULA

You often hear dieters talk about metabolism. That is because a slow metabolism means that the body is not burning many calories. Metabolism is the series of processes your body uses to function normally throughout the day, even when you are sleeping. If you make your metabolism work faster, you can burn more calories. The more calories you can burn, the greater your ability to lose weight. Sounds pretty simple, right?

It all depends on the kind of fuel you're filling up with. Those muscle cells are hungry little machines that want premium fuel. When you consider all the foods possible, it boils down to three key metabolism-maximizing nutrients that are the backbone of this program:

Protein + Vitamin C + Fiber

On the Feed Muscle, Shrink Fat program, every meal and snack will include these three key nutrients. It is the perfect formula for feeding muscle cells, shrinking fat cells, and losing weight.

Protein

Protein is the most important nutritional element for molding your body into the shape you desire. Proteins are broken down by the body into amino acids, the "building blocks of life." Proteins repair and rebuild muscle tissues, grow hair and nails, create enzymes and hormones, and maintain the health of internal organs and blood. Your body also needs protein to break down fat. Just as water provides transport, so does protein. Together, protein and water are extremely important for transporting fat for weight loss. In order for fat cells to open their doors and let the fat out to be burned as fuel, protein and water must be handy.

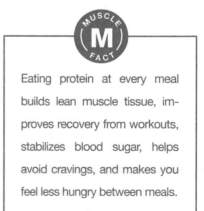

Eating protein at every meal builds lean muscle tissue, improves recovery from workouts, stabilizes blood sugar, helps avoid cravings, and makes you feel less hungry between meals.

Specifically protein consists of 22 amino acids. Eight are "essential," meaning that your body cannot manufacture them sufficiently or at all. It has to get them from the foods you eat. The others can be made by your body but are also found in food.

Protein supports weight loss because it causes you to feel full, making it much easier to leave the table. This is partly due to how much effort it takes your body to break down and utilize protein. It is work (and work means energy) for your body to divide proteins into amino acids that are absorbed and transported by the blood to cells for use. So the mere act of breaking down protein is burning calories and keeping your blood sugar stabilized in the process. Foods high in protein also help you feel full because they usually contain fat as well. The combination of fat and protein can keep you less hungry between meals.

Because protein is necessary to build and repair muscles, it is critical that you have a sufficient intake of protein to improve recovery from workouts. Without it not only will you feel low on energy and experience more muscle soreness, but you will also increase your risk for injury.

Vitamin C

Vitamin C is another key in the weight loss formula. Recent research suggests that you might be more successful at weight loss if you eat more fruits and vegetables high in vitamin C. According to a 2006 study at Arizona State University, individuals consuming sufficient amounts of vitamin C oxidize (burn) 30 percent *more* fat during moderate exercise than those who consume insufficient amounts. Too little vitamin C in the bloodstream was shown to correlate with increased body fat and waist measurements.

In another study published in 2003 at the University of Colorado at Boulder, researchers showed that taking more vitamin C may help older adults combat oxidative stress in their cells that may damage tissues and interfere with normal physiological functions. "Oxidative stress" is what happens when destructive molecules buddy up with oxygen in the body and hinder normal functions, some of which lead to lowered resting metabolisms. The Colorado study demonstrated that one group's metabolisms burned an average of almost 100 additional calories per day after an infusion of vitamin C directly into the veins.

Vitamin C is by no means a wonder drug for weight loss. But the reason I designed my program with a spotlight on this essential vitamin is clear: When you seek good sources of vitamin C, you find the highest-quality foods that offer a host of health benefits. The standard American diet is so stuffed with processed foods that many of us lack a sufficient supply of necessary vitamins and minerals. A report published in the *Journal of the American College of Nutrition* in 2005 notes that one in five Americans is vitamin C depleted and an additional 12 to 17 percent are vitamin C deficient. The report indicates that adults ages 25 to 44 have

All Calories Are Not Created Equal

In theory a calorie is a calorie. But does that mean there is no difference between eating 1,500 calories' worth of candy bars and 1,500 calories of turkey on rye? Absolutely not.

The body responds differently to calories from different sources. A candy bar loaded with refined sugar and unhealthy fat will likely be stored in your fat cells. There is not much (if any) protein in the candy to nourish muscles and boost metabolism. Plus candy causes insulin surges with every bite. By contrast the body must expend energy to break down protein and healthy fats found in the turkey on rye. That meal will provide balance throughout the day, stabilizing blood sugar and supplying a steady source of energy without insulin spikes.

the worst vitamin C levels. A full 18 percent of adults get fewer than 30 milligrams per day when the recommended allowance is a minimum of 75 for women and 90 for men. Some experts argue that the low-carb craze may be partly to blame as people push vitamin-C-rich fruits and vegetables aside.

Vitamin C is essential to the body's breakdown and utilization of food. The body can neither manufacture it nor store it. On the Feed Muscle, Shrink Fat plan, you will get crucial vitamin C from wholesome, nutrient-rich foods that will aid in your weight loss efforts and support your health. But if you want to take a supplement each day just to be sure your body is getting all of the necessary vitamins and minerals, that is perfectly fine. For more information about supplements and my list of personal recommendations, go to kathysmith.com.

Fiber

Science has proven fiber's many benefits: It improves heart health and can lower LDL (bad) cholesterol, blood pressure, and the risk for developing diabetes and some types of cancer. This is reason enough to love it, but there's more: Fiber keeps metabolism maximized. It allows the digestion of food to slow to a speed that supports muscle feeding and fat shrinking. It keeps you feeling fuller longer.

Let's explore this idea further. As I said before, timing is a key factor in what you eat. Because foods enter your bloodstream at different rates—some enter it in as little as five minutes, while others can take up to two hours—they change the chemistry of your hormones and either satiate you or stimulate you to want more.

If you eat a food that is high in simple carbohydrates and is quickly digested, it will enter your bloodstream quickly, causing a spike in insulin that is largely responsible for making you feel hungry for more.

Foods that satiate you take longer to get into your system, somewhere between 30 and 120 minutes. They help prevent insulin surges and maintain a healthy blood sugar balance. This ideal window of 30 to 120 minutes is created when you eat proteins and high-fiber vegetables, fruits, and grains. Because they take longer to enter your bloodstream, it actually requires more energy to break down. The body needs to process those protein and fat molecules and expend energy to do so, which is like exercise for the body without you physically moving. That is the science of food.

Fiber becomes a key player in creating a meal that will be digested slowly and is less likely to be converted to fat. Glucose in the presence of fiber will be released gradually into the bloodstream, providing continual bursts of energy over time while you're still feeling full. In fact you can combine a quickly digested food with a slowly digested one that has fiber and change the entire chemistry of a meal. Here is an example: Top a whole grain bagel or English muffin with peanut butter and a spoonful of flaxseed. The fat and fiber in the peanut butter and flaxseed will stop the glucose in the bagel from getting hurriedly digested.

Kathy's Secret: Fiber is a dieter's friend. Aim to eat at least 25 grams of fiber a day. Some studies suggest that consuming an extra 14 grams of fiber per day may cause the body to absorb 10 percent fewer calories.

Soluble Versus Insoluble Fiber

Fiber comes in two forms, soluble and insoluble. Soluble fiber dissolves in water and is found mostly in nuts, seeds, legumes (beans, lentils, peas), fruit, and oat bran. It is the "digestible" fiber that helps lower the risk for heart disease and can lower bad cholesterol. Insoluble fiber, on the other hand, does not dissolve in water, so it is the "indigestible" form. Found mostly in whole grains and vegetables, it acts like a rake through your system, pushing food along and aiding in digestive health. Do not worry whether you are getting soluble or insoluble fiber. On my program you will eat a balance of both to reap all the benefits.

THE IMPORTANCE OF FREQUENT MEALS

On the Feed Muscle, Shrink Fat plan, you will eat every three to four hours. This is critical for weight loss. We know now that grazers—those who nibble throughout the day rather than eat three big meals—have an easier time keeping weight down. That concept really hit home for me recently when I worked with a test group of women and men from around the country. Those who exercised consistently and ate balanced meals achieved weight loss results. But those who spaced meals evenly apart throughout the day achieved even greater success.

There is a reason why being famished does not feel good: The body does not like to operate low on fuel. It likes to be fed on a routine basis. By the same token you know the sensation of being absolutely stuffed is not all that great either.

The solution is to feel somewhere in between. That is what eating an ideal combination of food (protein + vitamin C + fiber) every three to four hours will accomplish. By spacing meals every three

The act of eating revs up the metabolism. It takes energy to digest food. On the Feed Muscle, Shrink Fat program, you'll be eating every 3 to 4 hours to keep your body's engines running at all times.

to four hours, you will avoid energy highs and lows that send metabolism on a roller coaster. It will keep metabolism revved, blood sugar levels constant, and insulin levels in check. Insulin is the hormone that ushers sugar out of the blood and into cells for use. (Or, if you overeat, excess sugar will be converted to fat.) Stabilizing insulin levels is a vital sign of health.

Simply knowing that you get to eat again in a few hours has important benefits. You won't have that "last meal" mentality that can lead to overeating. Spacing meals also helps preserve lean muscle mass. If you wait until you are starving, you tell your body to hold tightly onto fat to protect itself and to consume its muscle instead. Remember: Your muscles are your fat-burning machines. When you nourish muscle you maximize your body's allocation of energy and can deflate your fat cells. The more lean muscle mass you have, the more calories you will burn throughout the day and night. This has been proved time and time again in laboratory tests. In a weight loss study published in the *British Journal of Nutrition*, weight loss participants who ate frequent meals preserved considerably more lean muscle tissue than participants who ate fewer daily meals but consumed the same number of calories.

Typical Meal Frequency

Here is what a typical day on the Feed Muscle, Shrink Fat plan might look like:

Meal 1:   8 a.m.
Snack: 10:30 a.m.
Meal 2:   Noon
Snack: 3:30 p.m.
Meal 3:   7 p.m.

You don't have to follow this exact timeline; there are lots of other ways to create a schedule that works with your daily responsibilities. You should eat every three to four hours, but you can determine your specific hours. Here are some guidelines:

• You should eat within one hour of rising. So if you normally get up at 6 a.m., you should eat breakfast by 7 a.m. and then eat again around 10 a.m.

• Three mini meals (breakfast, lunch, and dinner) and two small snacks (one in midmorning and one in midafternoon) are ideal for keeping your energy level stable and your metabolism running.

Kathy's Secret: Some foods boosts your body's metabolism naturally while being digested and absorbed. Green tea is one such example, shown to potentially have metabolism-accelerating qualities. Hot peppers also have this effect.

• Avoid eating after 8 p.m. or within two hours of bedtime. At night our metabolism naturally slows down as our body prepares for sleep. If you eat too close to bedtime, you may have trouble falling asleep as the body (and digestion) tries to shut down and you have food in line to be processed. Late-night eating can be a pitfall for many, especially emotional eaters. Those who get bored can find themselves downing hundreds of extra calories when they really are not hungry. If you truly feel the need to eat something close to bedtime, go for a small snack (see page 43) or a cup of decaf herbal tea.

HOW EXERCISE MAXIMIZES FAT BURNING

It is common knowledge that exercise is great for you, and it is a key part of the Feed Muscle, Shrink Fat program. It can lower your risk for a multitude of diseases, including diabetes, cancer, heart disease, and osteoporosis. It helps you sleep better, improves your mood, staves off dementia in old age, and boosts immunity. You are probably aware that exercise helps you to burn more calories and lose weight more quickly. But you still might not understand why.

When you exercise and build muscles, you ultimately foster a stronger cardio-vascular system that pushes more oxygen through the body. A body with high oxygen levels is a body high on the me-tabolism meter. Metabolism increases as you are working out and can remain at an elevated state long afterward (called the "afterburn," which we will discuss more on page 85). This allows you to burn more calories and move fat out of cells for energy.

Exercise also helps you to maintain and build lean muscle mass, which you know by now is critical to your ability to burn fat. With a balance of cardio work and strength training, which you will do while on this program, you will increase

MUSCLE FACT

Men have 10 times more tes-tosterone than women. That is why men can build muscle more easily. Women are not likely to bulk up by virtue of their physiology. When women build muscle it shows up as a toned and sculpted physique.

your lean muscle mass to give yourself an even greater capacity to burn more calo-ries throughout the day and keep your metabolism running on high.

Success Story: Becky LaCroix

"I was 145 pounds before I got pregnant. During my pregnancy I got up to 184 pounds. I looked like a tank. Six weeks after giving birth, I started exercising for a wedding I was going to attend a few months later. With Kathy's program I lost 50 pounds and got down to 134 pounds for the wed-ding. But then I continued to lose weight. Now I am 129 pounds—even lighter than I was before I got preg-nant—all without "dieting."

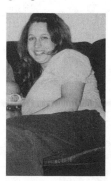
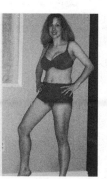

No, You Don't Have to Count Calories

On the Feed Muscle, Shrink Fat Diet, you don't have to count calories because I've done the calculations for you. I want this plan to be simple and uncomplicated, so I give you suggested portion sizes as guidelines instead of calorie counts. I want you to become so attuned to your body's needs and wishes, including its level of hunger and sense of fullness, that you can decide for yourself the proper portions for you without having to count calories, fat grams, or carbohydrates. But because people always ask about calories, here's the scoop.

Most women need a daily average of 1,500 to 1,800 calories; men need 1,600 to 2,200 calories. Of course this depends on activity levels, body size, and body type. The Feed Muscle, Shrink Fat plan includes three meals plus two snacks a day, for a total of 1,500 calories a day. Each meal is approximately 300 to 400 calories, and each snack is about 100 to 200 calories.

Because activity and hunger levels vary, I have built in plenty of flexibility in the Feed Muscle, Shrink Fat program so that you can tailor it to your needs. (See "Adjust Portion Sizes to Suit Your Needs," page 73.) However, during Week 1: Fast Track 1, you should follow my 1,500-calorie plan exactly as it is a realistic representation of what your body needs to function, make muscular gains, and shed body fat. As you move into Week 3 of the program, you will be able to make individual adjustments. This is when using your journal and logging on to my website for added support will be helpful.

WEEK 1: FAST TRACK 1

Now it is time to get started on the Feed Muscle, Shrink Fat program. Beginning today you are on your way to the best shape of your life!

RULES FOR FAST TRACK 1

During Week 1: Fast Track 1, you will follow my strict meal plan, which includes three meals and two snacks daily. I will tell you exactly what to eat from Day 1 to Day 7. Because you won't have to make any decisions about what to eat or when, you'll be able to focus on other important shifts you will make this week. Here are your Week 1: Fast Track 1 guidelines:

Rule 1: Follow the Meal Plans Exactly
Lean proteins and vegetables are the center of attention this week, and you are eliminating starchy carbohydrates, such as bread, pasta, rice, and cereal. (You will reincorporate them starting in Week 2.) Refined sugars and most sweets are off the list this week too, although you will be able to eat them in moderation later in the program. For your meals, follow the chart on page 45.

Rule 2: Eat Every Three to Four Hours
Remember, eating every three to four hours is critical to your success. Do not skip a meal or a snack. Eating frequently keeps your metabolism running in high gear, your blood sugar balanced, and your energy level maximized. You are less likely to feel either ravenous or painfully full, and you will stay satisfied between meals. Plus this continual intake of calories will eliminate those late-afternoon bonks.

Rule 3: Start Your Diary
If you haven't set up a journal yet, do it now. (For details on journal templates, see pages 81–82.) Be sure to record what you eat at every meal and snack and how much physical activity you're doing. Maintaining a journal will help you identify both good and unhealthy patterns in your eating habits. The journal also will help you stay motivated and on track by keeping you aware of what you are eating and what life events are affecting your mood, attitude, and behaviors.

Rule 4: Exercise for 10 Minutes

Starting on Day 1 you will do my revolutionary Matrix exercises for 10 minutes a day. Your exercise program starts on page 93. If this marks the first time in a while that you've engaged in physical activity, it is OK to go easy on yourself in the first couple of days. My hope is that you soon find that the rewards of exercise motivate you to adopt an active lifestyle forever. Exercise is so much more than a means to lose weight. It's how we stay young, healthy, spirited, and feeling in control. It should be nonnegotiable.

Rule 5: Stay Hydrated

Because hydration is key to weight loss and good health, you should drink at least six glasses of sugar-free liquids a day. At least five of those glasses should be water, which you should drink at every meal and snack.

If you normally drink caloric beverages like sugary soda and juices, you should make the shift to noncaloric varieties like water and unsweetened tea. A new study called "What America Drinks" reveals that on average Americans get 22 percent of their daily calories from nutrient-poor, sweetened beverages such as soft drinks, fruit-flavored drinks, and presweetened teas. Imagine what would happen if the average person simply switched from regular soda to water. She would cut 22 percent of the calories from her diet and shed pounds in a matter of weeks, even if she did nothing else!

Kathy's Secret: Bored with your drinks? Try Emergen-C®, a fizzy drink mix loaded with vitamins and minerals. It gives me a boost of energy and turns plain water into a refreshing, flavorful burst of supplements that helps the body run efficiently and boosts immunity. It comes in a variety of flavors and takes "hydration" to a whole new level.

There are many healthy drink options. Have decaf herbal tea as a morning beverage. To spruce up plain or carbonated water, add a slice of orange, lemon, lime, grapefruit, or even cucumber. Or simply brew your own tea (any kind you want) and chill it with ice. You should limit diet sodas to one or two cans each day because the artificial sweetener in sodas can make you crave sugary foods.

The skinny on alcohol. During Week 1: Fast Track 1 and Week 2: Fast Track 2, you should eliminate all alcohol. You will be able to reincorporate it back in Week 3. Remember, Fast Track 1 is meant to break old habits and recharge metabolism. Not only does alcohol have calories, but it can lower the defenses that keep us from overeating. So keep alcohol intake to a minimum.

The morning buzz. No, you don't have to quit drinking coffee or tea on the Feed Muscle, Shrink Fat plan. But you do need to evaluate your choices (record them in your journal) and maybe make a few modifications. Caffeine drinks can often hide a colossal amount of fat and calories, especially the designer blends that add cocoa and caramel. Even some tea concoctions have more to do with sugar and additives than traditional tea. Use the following guidelines when ordering your cup:

- Avoid drinks with heavy creams and sugary syrups.
- Choose drip coffees with "calorie-free" flavors, such as hazelnut, vanilla, and cinnamon.
- Opt for hot teas with lots of "free" flavors like jasmine, rosemary, chamomile, mint, cinnamon, and apple spice.
- Avoid caffeine after 3 p.m.
- Use a dollop of natural honey to sweeten a cup of hot tea. Sprinkle in one serving of raw sugar to sweeten iced tea.
- If you crave a fanciful blend, choose low-calorie concoctions that use nonfat milk and no added sugar.

Rule 6: Substitute Protein Shakes for Meals

For optimum results during Fast Track 1, I encourage you to substitute one of my nutritious power shakes for up to two meals a day. These delicious, easy-to-make shakes will help supercharge your weight loss for a reason you may not expect. They remove the temptation to "cheat" as you cook a meal, tasting a little here and a little there. Because they pack a perfect mix of protein, healthy fat, and carbs, they will give you lots of energy and keep you feeling satisfied. By mixing them into Fast Track 1, you will maximize results and put yourself on a faster track.

Shakes have been a part of my life for decades. You will find recipes for my seven favorites on pages 232–235, and I know you will love them as much as I do.

While they are extremely helpful during Fast Track 1 for keeping calories in check, feel free to substitute a shake for a meal whenever you like in the next six weeks. I regularly drink shakes because I just love how much energy and nutrition they provide without a lot of fuss. You will soon have these shake recipes memorized for whenever you want a pick-me-up or have a craving for something cold, smooth, and filling.

If you are accustomed to sugary-fruit smoothies and ice cream-based shakes, it may take time to get used to my blends, which include protein powder. Most grocery stores now carry protein powder. Make sure you don't buy "meal replacement" powder. Look for a brand that contains whey, egg whites, or soy and has a serving size of about 2 tablespoons or 100 calories. Feel free to play with the ingredients too. If you prefer icier blends over thicker ones, just add more ice, try frozen fruit instead of fresh, and mix in water instead of milk. Protein powders also come in flavors like vanilla, chocolate, and strawberry. You can mix these flavors in the recipes to your heart's desire.

Rule 7: Don't Forget to Snack

In Week 1: Fast Track 1, you should eliminate all starchy carbohydrates, including snacks such as crackers, bread, nuts, and nut butters. But you will still have plenty of snack options (see page 43). You can have two snacks a day—ideally, one in midmorning and one between lunch and dinner. The goal is to scatter your snacks between your meals so you are eating every three to four hours. If you go too long without eating, your metabolism will slow and you will arrive at your next meal so hungry that it will be difficult to control your portions. When your metabolism is slow, food is more easily stored as fat.

Rule 8: Indulge in Desserts

When do you get a real treat? Every day! There is a time and place for sneaking in a sugary indulgence at every step of the Feed Muscle, Shrink Fat program. After all, sweets can satisfy us in ways nothing else can. The problem with most sweets is they tend to be high in saturated fat and made with highly refined sugar that we are physically programmed to crave more of after a small bite. You know the experience. You say you will have just one cookie and then it becomes difficult to abstain from the next one and then the next one.

The following is a list of treats you can have during Fast Track 1 (limit one per day). This list will grow as your options open in Week 3.

- Diet Swiss Miss Hot Chocolate® or Carnation Hot Chocolate Light®
- Sugar-Free Jell-O® pudding or Sugar-Free Jell-O®
- 1 single Popsicle®, Fudgsicle®, or Creamsicle®
- The Skinny Cow Fat-Free Fudge Bar® or The Skinny Cow Ice Cream Sandwich®
- Weight Watchers Smart Ones Pop®
- ½ cup berries with 1 tablespoon Fat-Free Reddi-Wip®
- ½ cup berries with ½ cup nonfat vanilla yogurt with ¼ ounce shaved dark chocolate on top (This is one of my all-time favorites!)
- ½ grapefruit sprinkled with stevia or Splenda®
- 1 ounce dark chocolate (Tip: Go for chocolate that has 60 percent or more cocoa. It is higher in healthful antioxidants.)
- Cup of tea with a teaspoon of honey or agave nectar

SNACK ATTACKS

Enjoy any of these snack options once a day during the six-week Feed Muscle, Shrink Fat program.

Celery sticks with 1 to 1½ tablespoons soy nut butter, almond butter, or natural crunchy peanut butter
Bell peppers, sliced, with 2 triangles of Laughing Cow® light cheese smeared inside
Starkist® tuna (5-ounce bag) wrapped in lettuce leaves (optional: dress up the tuna with dillweed, lemon juice, green onions, light mayo, and/or lemon pepper)
2 seaweed wraps with 2 ounces light cheese and 4 ounces turkey slices
2 hard-cooked egg whites, cauliflower, or celery dipped in 1 to 1½ tablespoons hummus
1 hard-cooked egg, sliced and served with diced tomatoes or salsa
1 green apple with 1 ounce (1 slice) low-fat or string cheese
2 ounces turkey, beef, or salmon jerky with ½ or 1 medium cucumber
1 cup sugar snap peas with 1 ounce Jarlsberg light cheese
¾ cup plain low-fat or fat-free yogurt (preferably organic) with ½ cup berries
½ cup low-fat or fat-free cottage cheese with ½ cup berries, kiwi, or cantaloupe
¾ cup edamame (soybeans)
1 to 2 tablespoons ricotta, feta, or hummus with celery sticks or bell peppers
4 asparagus stalks wrapped with 4 ounces turkey slices (optional: add mustard)
1 hard-cooked egg with balsamic vinegar and steamed asparagus or spinach
½ cup low-fat cottage cheese and salsa
1 wedge (¼ of 1 whole) cantaloupe with ½ cup low-fat or fat-free cottage cheese
2 to 3 ounces roasted turkey with ¼ avocado rolled up inside (optional: add mustard)
1 cup plain low-fat or fat-free cottage cheese sprinkled with cinnamon and nutmeg and ½ chopped apple
½ cup low-fat or fat-free cottage cheese and steamed green beans
1 high-fiber bar (look for one that has less than 200 calories, at least 5 grams of fiber, and fewer than 20 grams of sugar)
Cucumber Boats (see recipes, pages 228–229)
Asparagus Wrap-Ups (see recipe, page 226)
Edamame Salad (see recipe, page 227)
Not Your Mother's Onion Dip (see recipe, page 226)
Parmesan Crisps with Smoked Turkey (see recipe, page 227)

Kathy's Secret: If you've already had your dessert for the day but you're still craving something sugary, here's my surefire way to kill a sweet tooth: Drink tart cranberry juice. I like to mix 1 ounce of unsweetened cranberry juice with 7 ounces of water. The calories are negligible so this little trick doesn't count as a snack.

A caution about sugar substitutes. Many of the reduced- or low-calorie desserts you see in the grocery store are made with artificial sweeteners. Although some sweeteners, such as aspartame and saccharin, are 100 percent artificial, some—such as Splenda®—are made from real sugar.

Personally I don't like using artificial sweeteners and prefer to use real, natural sugar when I need to sweeten something. Artificial sweetners can be a double-edged sword. Yes, they can help cut calories while providing sweetness, but they also can mess with your body's chemistry that helps you control how much you eat. Artificial sweeteners may trigger intense cravings. It is up to you to decide whether you want to continue eating artificial sugars based on how your body responds to them. You may want to try an experiment by avoiding them entirely for a week or two to see how you feel. Instead of sprinkling your berries with a packet of Equal®, try a teaspoon of real sugar, honey, or agave nectar.

When to Repeat Fast Track 1

Fast Track 1 is so effective at helping you shed fat quickly and safely that you may want to use it for two weeks in a row. Simply repeat the meal and exercise plan, then proceed to Fast Track 2 (see page 47).

Use it any time you need to drop a few pounds in a short time. You can even use Fast Track for just a day to recalibrate your blood sugar and charge your metabolism if you have not been eating healthfully and exercising.

Because it is such a strict regimen, you should not use Fast Track 1 for more than two weeks in a row. If you stay on Fast Track 1 for too long, you may eventually succumb to intense cravings for off-limits foods, specifically starchy carbohydrates and sweets.

MEAL PLAN WEEK 1: FAST TRACK 1

Meals: For optimum results during Week 1, substitute one or two of the meals with a protein shake using any of the recipes on pages 232–235.
Vegetables: During Week 1, when the menu lists "with a vegetable" choose any vegetable recipe in the "Sides" section (starting on page 218) except for those containing zucchini and squash (which are too starchy for Week 1).
Snacks: You can choose up to two snacks each day.

Day 1	
Breakfast	Asparagus Baked Frittata (page 186)
Lunch	Farmer's Market Chopped Salad (page 193)
Dinner	Tipapia With Greens (page 209) with a vegetable
Day 2	
Breakfast	Garden Omelet (page 184)
Lunch	Quick-Fix Salad (page 192)
Dinner	Grilled Chicken Breasts or Turkey Cutlets (page 214) with a vegetable
Day 3	
Breakfast	Quick-Fix Egg Scramble (page 181)
Lunch	Blue Plate Turkey Burger Salad (page 196)
Dinner	New Orleans Halibut (page 207) with a vegetable
Day 4	
Breakfast	Gazpacho Sundae (page 166)
Lunch	Mediterranean Chicken Wrap-Ups (page 188)
Dinner	Asian Glazed Salmon (page 208) with a vegetable
Day 5	
Breakfast	Kathy's Yogurt Sundae (page 165)
Lunch	Tuscan Bean and Tuna Salad (page 197)
Dinner	Fish in a Packet (page 209) with a vegetable
Day 6	
Breakfast	2 eggs (any style) with steamed asparagus and 2 pieces turkey bacon or sausage OR 1 cup cottage cheese
Lunch	Grilled chicken breast with a vegetable
Dinner	Chicken Skewers (page 204) with a vegetable
Day 7	
Breakfast	Western-Style Omelet (page 183)
Lunch	Niçoise Roll-Ups (page 190)
Dinner	Tuscan Chicken (page 203) with a vegetable

Week 1: Fast Track 1 Summary

✴ Eat three meals + two snacks a day.

✴ Eat every three to four hours.

✴ Avoid starchy carbohydrates, sugars, nuts, and salt.

✴ Drink at least six glasses of sugar-free liquid a day (at least five of the six glasses should be water).

✴ Substitute a protein shake for one or two meals.

Success Story: Mary Morgan

"I have lost more than 30 inches across my body and a total of 27 pounds, and I just feel fantastic! It's a wonderful feeling to have this kind of confidence in my body. I feel very fit, very tight. I've got killer abs right now that I really have a great time showing off! You don't realize how big the transformation is until you see it boldly in front if you! I can't imagine anybody not succeeding with this program."

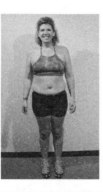
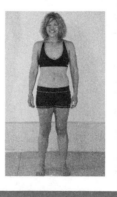

Photos provided by Beachbody.com

WEEK 2: FAST TRACK 2

Fast Track 1 gave you discipline, broke some bad habits, motivated you, weaned you from cravings, and generally jumpstarted your fat-burning engines. Now it's time for Fast Track 2, when you incorporate more carbohydrates into your diet. You will follow the same rules as in Fast Track 1—stick to the meal plan, eat every three to four hours, drink lots of water, write in your diary, and exercise. But you will make a few more shifts as well.

RULES FOR FAST TRACK 2

Rule 1: Add Carbs and Starchy Grains

You will continue to eat three meals and two snacks a day, but you'll bring back grains and starchy carbohydrates, such as breads, pastas, rice, and potatoes. During Fast Track 2 I have again taken away all the guesswork by giving you a week's worth of great-tasting, fresh meals. You will find the meal plan on page 50; the corresponding recipes start on page 163. These easy-to-prepare meals will help you train your body to feel satisfied with the perfect calorie load for you.

Despite what you may have heard about recent diet crazes and fads, carbohydrates are critical for supplying energy, building muscle, keeping you full, and fueling your brain. The right starches also are necessary for successful weight loss. The fact is that if you are not getting enough carbs, your body will turn to muscle for energy, breaking it down and converting its protein molecules to glucose for much-needed fuel. While it can use fat for energy in the absence of any glucose or glycogen (stored glucose), it is easier for the body to resort to muscle. This pushes you in the wrong direction. To avoid this muscle-wasting, fat-paralysis state, you need to have a steady intake of starchy carbohydrates in your diet.

There are many healthy carbohydrates from which to choose on the Feed Muscle, Shrink Fat plan, and they deserve special attention because everyone responds differently to them. Some carbs can trigger reactions in your body that can work against your weight loss goals and, ultimately, your overall health. I will teach you the common guidelines for choosing healthy carbs, and you will tune in to how you feel after eating them. You will quickly catch on to which carbs you should eat frequently, which you should eat occasionally, and which you should eat rarely.

Rule 2: Be Flexible

You have more options to be creative with your meals in Fast Track 2. You can eat any meal from Fast Track 1. Or mix up the days in Fast Track 2 and eat Wednesday's lunch on Monday, for instance. In addition I welcome you to try a recipe from one of my hometown restaurants starting this week. You will find them in "Kathy's California Restaurant Favorites," starting on page 240.

Rule 3: Have Patience with Your Weight Loss

Fast Track 2 is a stabilizing week, so your weight loss may not be as rapid as in Fast Track 1. But by now you have built a foundation for the kind of weight loss that lasts a lifetime. It is steady and healthy, and you won't feel lethargic or moody as you continue your journey because you will enjoy luscious, energy-supplying power foods from many food categories. You also will gain a heightened appreciation for the foods that boost your metabolism, give you sustained energy for exercise and optimum performance, keep you deeply satisfied, and render a new, vibrant you.

Rule 4: Snack Every Day

As you know by now, eating every three to four hours is key to your weight loss success. Snacks help keep your metabolism revved so you are constantly burning energy. They also factor into maintaining blood sugar balance, sustaining feelings of fullness, and nourishing those muscles. You can continue to have two snacks a day. Choose anything from the Fast Track 1 list (page 43). You also may add the following snack options to your choices this week:

- 1 ounce low-fat cheese or 1 tablespoon soft goat cheese on 5 whole grain crackers
- 15 to 20 almonds with jicama slices
- 8 to 10 almonds with a small pear
- A small handful (8 to 12) mixed raw nuts: almonds, peanuts, walnuts, and cashews
- 1 tablespoon nut butter with 5 whole grain crackers or 1 slice whole grain toast

Rule 5: Indulge in Desserts

Choose from the same list of desserts as in Fast Track 1 (page 42). Next week you will begin to prepare more elaborate desserts using my recipes.

Rule 6: Learn to Season Without Salt

Even if you buy a simple can of sliced carrots at the store, you are getting more than just carrots. You're probably also getting preservatives and one of the biggest additives in food processing—salt. I know some of us get excited sometimes when we find a food that has few or no calories, like canned olives or pickles, but you can't forget to look at that sodium content per serving. Sodium is directly linked to a number of health issues, including high blood pressure and heart disease. It also can cause water retention that makes you bloated and uncomfortable. (Ironically drinking water can come to the rescue here. It will encourage your cells to release sodium that is causing the bloat.) A great rule of thumb is if the milligrams of sodium per serving is greater than the calories per serving, you should consider that product high in sodium.

Instead of grabbing the salt shaker, use alternative spices and herbs. Experiment with different brands and blends until you find one tailored to your palate. The following have big flavors that take quick dishes to a new level of satisfaction without adding fat or preservatives:

SALT SUBSTITUTES

Adding salt is not the only way to enhance the flavor of your meals. Try any of these substitutions to add tremendous flavor without increasing the sodium level.

Dillweed	Use in rice and fish dishes.
Leaves (basil, mint, etc.)	Use with eggs, seafood, chicken, cucumbers, green beans, potatoes, tomatoes, and beets.
Garlic	Shake garlic powder onto salads, meat, fish, poultry, and into dressings. Chop fresh garlic to use in recipes.
Oregano	It is a classic with meat, fish, poultry, eggs, vegetable soup, and eggplant.
Saffron	It adds full flavor to fish soups, stews, and breads.
Tarragon	Use it sparingly at first for zing on chicken, fish, shellfish, and carrots and in dressings.
Salt-free Italian seasoning	Add it to boiling pasta water for an Italian accent.
Fresh lemon juice	Squeeze it on steamed vegetables, broiled fish, rice, or pasta.
Salt-free garlic and herb seasoning	Use it to liven up soups, sandwiches, or your home-cooked meals.

MEAL PLAN WEEK 2: FAST TRACK 2

Meals: Don't forget you can choose any meal from Week 1.
Vegetables: Choose any vegetable as a side from the list of recipes on page 63. You can also add back zucchini and squash.
Snacks: You can have up to 2 snacks per day.

Day 1	
Breakfast	Mexican-Style Scramble (page 178)
Lunch	Curried Chicken Salad in Papaya (page 192)
Dinner	Broiled Salmon Dijonnaise (page 208) with a vegetable
Day 2	
Breakfast	Hawaiian Crunch (page 165)
Lunch	Tuscan Bean and Tuna Salad (page 197)
Dinner	Chili-Rubbed Chicken Breasts with Mango Salsa (page 202) and a vegetable
Day 3	
Breakfast	Quick-Fix Waffle Breakfast (page 173)
Lunch	Niçoise Roll-Ups (page 190)
Dinner	Master Stir-Fry (page 213)
Day 4	
Breakfast	Berry-Oatmeal Crunch (page 168)
Lunch	Thai Beef Salad (page 198)
Dinner	Turkey Meatballs Marinara (page 206) over pasta
Day 5	
Breakfast	Quick-Fix Cereal (page 169)
Lunch	Popeye Burgers (page 189) with a quick-fix salad (no meat added)
Dinner	Tilapia Saute with Greens (page 209) and a vegetable
Day 6	
Breakfast	Sausage Sandwich (page 174)
Lunch	Quick-Fix Sandwich (page 189) with a vegetable
Dinner	Fish in a Packet (page 209) with a vegetable
Day 7	
Breakfast	Italian-Style Scramble (page 177) plus 2 pieces turkey bacon or sausage or 1 cup low-fat cottage cheese
Lunch	Chinese Chicken Salad (page 194)
Dinner	Steamed Fish with Chinese Herbs (page 207) and a vegetable

Week 2: Fast Track 2 Summary

✳ Eat three meals + two snacks a day.

✳ Eat every three to four hours.

✳ Reintroduce healthy carbohydrates such as breads, pasta, and rice.

✳ Continue to drink at least six glasses of sugar-free liquid a day (at least five of the six glasses should be water).

✳ Snack at least twice a day with expanded options.

✳ Exercise six times a week.

✳ Be patient if weight loss slows this week.

Success Story: Linette Rubio

"Before I found Kathy Smith, I had no self-confidence and didn't care about fixing myself at all. I often didn't even do my hair or makeup. Then I started doing Kathy's program and it gave me so much con-

fidence. I lost 27 pounds and went from 28 percent body fat down to 15.7 percent. I'm so happy with the way I look, and I even feel good enough to wear a bathing suit now."

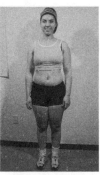
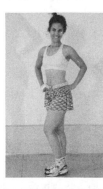

Photos provided by Beachbody.com

WEEKS 3–6: MAXIMUM FAT BURN

As you enter Week 3, your body already has begun to change. In addition to being lighter, you may notice that your cravings have weakened, you don't want to binge on high-fat, salty foods, and you can better regulate your appetite. Your energy levels are higher, your mind is sharper, and you sleep better. You have evened out your blood sugar levels, maximized your metabolism, and turned your body into a fat-shrinking machine. I also hope that my recipes have given you a taste for how wonderful wholesome food can be and that my exercise plan has you addicted to the pleasures of movement. As you fall in love with the new you, chances are you won't want to go back to your old, unhealthy ways. The work you did in the previous two weeks has prepared you for continued weight loss and lifelong weight management. You already have begun to make the lifestyle changes that will usher in vibrant health and support continued weight loss.

RULES FOR MAXIMUM FAT BURN

Once again you will build on the habits and lifestyle shifts you've made in the last two weeks. You will continue to eat three meals a day plus two snacks.

Rule 1: Design Your Own Meals

If the first two weeks felt too restrictive because I told you exactly what to eat, now you can broaden your options and have more flexibility. Starting in Week 3 you can plan your daily meals by using my recipes and planned meals or by improvising your own meals following my simple guidelines that are based on the simple Feed Muscle, Shrink Fat formula: lean proteins + vitamin C + fiber. (It's easy with my Plate Method, which you'll read about on page 58.) The choice is up to you. Of course you also can do a mixture of both—design some of your own meals and occasionally rely on mine. By this point in the program, you already have changed the way you relate to nutrition. This is when you end your need for a "diet" and you become an independent, healthy eater.

Granted, new lifestyle habits take time and practice to become second nature, and that is why I'm going to continue to help you build your meals this week by taking you step-by-step through the process of choosing the right proteins, vegetables, grains, and complementing fats.

If you can learn how to incorporate every food you ever want in your diet without derailing your weight loss goals and health needs, then that is what I call success. So I'm going to show you how to have some of your favorite family meals, including meats, pastas, and desserts that deliver a healthy dose of good nutrition. The recipes you used in the past two weeks should have clued you in to how easy this can be.

Rule 2: Eat Every Three to Four Hours

This rule is worth repeating. If you found it challenging to have your meals every three to four hours during the last two weeks (and you will know this by looking at your diary), try to schedule them better starting this week. By training yourself to eat every three to four hours, you will be able to control your portions much better. You not only will see far greater weight loss results but will also feel better. You'll have more energy and mental clarity. You will feel light and alive, and that will allow you to accomplish a lot more in your workouts and beyond.

Many people think they don't have time to eat this often. Or they find time only to grab some fast food or pick up a packaged meal that is heavy on calories and light on nutrition. But you know from the first two weeks that there are lots of ways to whip up a healthy meal quickly or create a grab-and-go meal or snack. You don't have to spend a lot of time in the kitchen.

Rule 3: Exercise

This week your activity level increases. You will find your Matrix instructions starting on page 85, as well as ideas for taking your fitness routine to new heights.

Rule 4: Be Patient with Weight Loss

If you lost more than 8 pounds in the first two weeks, then don't be discouraged if your weight loss slows. This is to be expected and is part of the normal weight loss process. Those first two weeks played a significant role in your overall weight loss efforts. They recalibrated your body, got your metabolism poised to lose more fat weight and gain lean muscle mass, and helped dampen cravings.

Keep in mind that during Week 2, you reintroduced starchier carbs into your diet, and your body held more water as a result. This also is common and part of your body's normal process as it begins to shed fat weight and optimize its burn capacity in terms of a fast metabolism. You also are gaining muscle from your workouts, which naturally adds more weight because muscle is heavier than fat. So while you may think you are regaining fat, the opposite is true: You are increasing your fat-shrinking muscle, which will transform your body in the long run.

Be patient with yourself during these final four weeks. Start paying more attention to how you *feel* and how your clothes fit as opposed to what the scale reads. It is highly unlikely that you are hitting a plateau at this point, but your body is going through lots of physical and chemical changes.

Rule 5: Learn to Wine and Dine

You will be able to add alcohol to your diet this week. (You should avoid it during Weeks 1 and 2.) Although alcohol is composed mainly of sugar alcohols, these are not metabolized in exactly the same way as sugars. But they still contain significant amounts of carbohydrate calories that inhibit the body's ability to burn fat. Most alcohol doesn't contain actual fat (exceptions include creamy liqueurs and coconut or chocolate blends). But because the body can't process and eliminate many alcohols at one time, their calories are rapidly converted and stored as fat, usually landing right in the lower belly as an unwanted paunch or roll.

Nevertheless, just like sensible carb eating, there is a way to drink smartly. Here are some tips:

- **Never drink alcohol on an empty stomach.** Always pair an alcoholic beverage with a protein to help stabilize blood sugar. A smart snack, for example, could be a 4-ounce glass of wine with slices of turkey and bell peppers.
- **Limit your intake of starch when you drink alcohol.** When you decide to indulge in an alcoholic drink, delete a starch (bread, pasta, etc.).
- **Alternate with water.** For every alcoholic beverage you have, drink 8 ounces of water. This helps keep you full and staves off a headache the next day.
- **Watch the ingredients.** Avoid alcoholic beverages mixed with sugary ingredients such as fruit juices, syrups, and regular soda. The calories add up: One ounce of 80-proof alcohol contains about 90 calories—before mixers are added. Even tonic water has 125 calories per 12 ounces! Instead use a twist of lime or lemon, diet soda, sparkling water, seltzer, or club soda.
- **Choose red.** Instead of spirits, beer, and white wine, opt for red wine, which contains some nutrients and antioxidants.

Rule 6: Use Your Journal and Go Online for Support

Use your journal to record what you eat, when, and how you feel after every meal. Remember to visit kathysmith.com for downloadable journal pages (or see pages 81–82). Make a note, for example, if you find it hard to stop eating a certain food because it triggers an endless sense of hunger. If a meal's portion doesn't satisfy you, make note of that too. Record your daily activities as well so you can look for emerging patterns and habits you may want to change.

SAMPLE MEALS WEEK 3–6: FAT BURN

Below is a sample menu for a day, including three main meals and two small snacks. I list where you get your proteins and produce and then add grains and dairy twice a day.

Meal 1 (about 7 a.m.): Egg white scramble with tomatoes, spinach, avocado. Plus toast.	
Protein:	4 egg whites (complementing fat: ¼ avocado [chopped])
Produce:	1 chopped tomato, 1 cup packed fresh spinach leaves
Grain:	1 slice whole grain toast
Extras:	chopped cilantro, salt and pepper to taste

Snack 1 (about 10:30 a.m.): Red Berry Sunrise Shake (recipe, page 232)

Meal 2 (about 1:30 p.m.): Grilled Chicken Salad (recipe, page 191)	
Protein:	4 ounces skinless chicken breast (complementing fat: 1 tablespoon olive oil in balsalmic-based dressing)
Produce:	4 cups mixed salad greens with chopped celery, cucumber, and cherry tomatoes
Grain:	(no grain)

Snack 2 (about 4:30 p.m.): 1 cup fat-free vanilla yogurt with ½ cup mixed berries and 4 crushed walnuts

Meal 3 (about 7:30 p.m.): Grilled salmon with asparagus and brown rice	
Protein:	4 ounces wild salmon (no fat added because this is a high-fat protein)
Produce:	10 stalks of steamed asparagus
Grain:	½ cup brown rice

After-dinner treat: ½ cup fresh strawberries and fat-free Reddi-Wip with ¼ ounce grated dark chocolate sprinkled on top

Target totals for the day:
- 4 to 6 servings of proteins (a "serving" is 3 to 6 ounces)
- 3 to 8 servings of vegetables/fruit
- 2 grains
- 2 dairies

Weeks 3–6: Maximum Fat Burn Summary

✳ Eat three meals + two snacks a day.

✳ Eat every three to four hours.

✳ Follow the Plate Method (see page 58) to design healthy meals.

✳ Eat healthy carbohydrates.

✳ Drink at least six glasses of sugar-free liquid a day (at least five of the six glasses should be water).

✳ For convenience substitute a protein shake for one meal.

✳ Reintroduce alcohol this week, if desired.

✳ Push yourself harder when exercising.

✳ Set the stage for burning fat and building muscle.

DESIGNING YOUR MEALS

Food is a source of profound pleasure. I love the crunch of an apple, the texture and smell of warm bread, the savory taste of roasted chicken. I delight in the cool sweetness of ice cream and the absolute ecstasy of chocolate cake. I cherish the meals my family and I share in our kitchen as much as I do great meals prepared in restaurants. I love food, and I love to eat.

What I have learned about food reflects what I have learned about life: Food has to be both functional and flexible. It has to meet my nutritional needs while allowing my choices to vary day to day. The same goes for you too. While it is certainly OK to have your own set of guidelines to follow, they needn't be extremely rigid and unyielding. Don't choose food just because you think it is "good for you" when you really don't like it. What fun is that?

Choose foods based on how they serve you physically, mentally, and emotionally. You can become a "functional" eater by learning to assess your needs at any given moment and how to decide what to eat based on those needs. This is something most of us are not used to doing. Either we get lazy and don't want to think about what we eat or we go on an unrealistic diet that tells us exactly what to eat.

Consistency is not about rigidity. If you do "slip," all you do is get back on track as soon as possible. Eventually you find yourself slipping less and less. When you blend consistency with flexibility, you achieve a truly functional approach to food and eating. You learn how to incorporate food into your life in a way that makes sense for your body and the way you live.

Remember, the Feed Muscle, Shrink Fat plan is based on my science-supported formula for healthy weight loss:

Protein + Vitamin C + Fiber = Weight Loss

These are the ingredients your body craves for optimum health. Commit this equation to memory to help you choose the superfoods that will fuel muscles, shrink fat, and boost your overall health. I will teach you how to identify the foods that contain these essential ingredients. Once you know that, what to eat becomes second nature.

As you're about to learn, lean proteins, wholesome vegetables, and nonstarchy grains will be your staples at virtually every meal. These are the foods that lie at the heart of the Feed Muscle, Shrink Fat blueprint. I will help you choose the right foods so you learn to design nutritious, delicious meals. This program is all about being satisfied, and there is no room for deprivation.

THE PLATE METHOD

Now that you are on your own and ready to design your own meals, I want you to think of the Plate Method when deciding what type of foods and how much of them to eat. With today's jumbo restaurant portions and supersize snacks, it is often difficult to recognize what is indeed a proper "serving." The Plate Method is a simple way to ensure that each of your meals is balanced and has the right portion sizes. All you have to do is visually split your plate into three parts.

Section 1: Protein
The first section of your plate is for protein (for example, turkey, fish, chicken, or lean beef). The right portion of protein will be about the size of a deck of cards or the palm of your hand. Protein and veggies are what stabilize your blood sugar and keep you satisfied.

Section 2: Fruits and Nonstarchy Veggies
This section of your plate gives you that important vitamin C. You can load your plate with as many leafy vegetables like spinach, asparagus, or green salad as you want. This is one section where it is OK to fill up! Because some fruits contain concentrated sugars, you will need to pace yourself better and go easy on these.

Section 3: Whole Grains
The third section of the plate is reserved for complex carbohydrates in the form of whole grains such as brown rice. I have included starchy vegetables like potatoes, yams, and corn in this category. Starting in Week 3 you will add grains/starchy vegetables to two meals each day. Keep your servings to about the size of a single scoop of ice cream.

You will create your meals within the Plate Method, then "add on" dairy, fats, and desserts. These add-ons are important because they deliver more nutrition and calories. This may sound counterproductive, but you need to be sure your caloric intake doesn't dip too low. It is not ideal to lose more than two pounds a week, especially during this Fat Burn phase, because the body can't adjust to rapid changes in chemistry. Therefore, you will "add on" one or two servings of dairy plus two fruits a day. Limit your fat intake at each meal to about the size of your thumb.

Having a sense of an ideal portion for your body's needs is the key to weight loss. It also will allow you to finish a meal feeling satisfied and full of energy. Who doesn't want that?

CHOOSING PROTEINS

Proteins play a key role in your ability to lose weight, plus they help satiate you, build muscle mass, and boost metabolism. In short, proteins feed your muscles so you can shrink your fat. It doesn't get much simpler than that. But Americans don't get the right proteins—or the right amounts. Most people eat far more protein than they need and from sources like steak and cheese that are loaded with saturated fat. Other people buy foods on the run that they may think are protein sources but in reality have more starchy carbs and unhealthy fats than lean, nutritious protein.

Eating the proper balance of healthy carbohydrates and fat with protein is essential. If your body gets deprived of much-needed fuel, it can find quick sources by literally feasting on (breaking down) muscle mass. That is why you should always incorporate muscle-feeding protein into your meals and even into your snacks.

Best Bets

There is a simple solution: low-fat, high-protein foods. With all the extra-lean meats available, it is easy to buy protein without all the fat. Turkey, chicken, eggs, most fish, and soy-based proteins are the best sources for high-quality, low-fat protein, whereas red meats, duck, and pork are higher in fat and should be limited in portion size. (See chart, page 61.) It is OK to have 4 to 5 ounces of lean chicken, but reduce your serving to only 3 or 4 ounces of sirloin steak. Eat medium- to high-fat proteins only twice a week. These include higher-fat fish, chicken thighs, eggs with yolks, turkey sausage or bacon, and red meats.

Vegetable Sources

Instead of getting your protein from meat, try vegetable sources, which come packed with complex carbohydrates plus protein. The richest sources of vegetable protein are legumes—dried peas and beans, including lentils, black-eyed peas, soybeans, kidney beans, pinto beans, and black beans.

All About Fish

Salmon and other types of cold-water fish contain heart-healthy omega-3 fatty acids. But you are probably aware that high levels of mercury, polychlorinated biphenyls (PCBs), and other pollutants have been measured in all sorts of fish from different parts of the world. So are fish healthy or harmful? Do the benefits of eating fish outweigh the potential risks associated with the alleged toxins? While there is no definitive answer on just how harmful these contaminants are, it is wise to take the reports into consideration and be mindful of where we get our fish and how much of it we eat. So I recommend two things: First, consume cold-water fish like salmon two or three times a week, and second, seek wild, not farmed, varieties. Speak with your local grocer in the seafood department for ideas on selecting the best and freshest types of fish. You may have to spend a little more money for wild seafood, but it is worth it. You will find these fish more flavorful too.

How Much Protein Do You Need?
It depends on your body size and activity level. For an active adult the Recommended Dietary Allowance (RDA) for protein is 0.36 gram per 1 pound of body weight. For a 150-pound woman, that equals 54 grams. Different foods contain different amounts of protein. Most of the foods listed in the chart on page 61 have about 7 grams per ounce.

It is OK to eat more protein than the RDA. Because the Feed Muscle, Shrink Fat program strives to build and maintain lean muscle mass while boosting activity levels, my meal plans and suggestions call for slightly more protein than the RDA standards, which are a bare minimum.

Protein Needs and Vegetarians
If you are a vegetarian or get most of your protein from plant sources, you must choose your protein sources carefully. Meat, chicken, fish, eggs, and milk products contain all of the essential amino acids. However, the protein in most plant sources is "incomplete," meaning it is missing one or another amino acid. You can easily rectify this by combining two incomplete proteins that complement each other. You don't need to eat complementary proteins in the same meal, just a variety of different protein sources on a regular basis. Here are some combinations that will work:
- Rice and beans or sesame seeds
- Wheat and nut butters
- Beans with wheat or corn

SMART PROTEIN OPTIONS

	Low-Fat Proteins *Eat 4 to 5 ounces at any given meal.*	Medium- to High-Fat Proteins *Limit to 3 to 4 ounces two times a week. Try to eat fish 2 to 3 times a week.*
Poultry		
	turkey breast, no skin	turkey sausage
	chicken breast, no skin	mixed white/dark chicken, no skin
		chicken leg with skin
		chicken thigh
		duck
		turkey hot dog
Fish		
	shrimp	halibut
	shellfish, crab	swordfish
	tuna in water	trout
	orange roughy	sea bass
	flounder	mahi mahi
	cod, sole	snapper, perch
		yellowtail
		salmon
Soy		
		1 cup soybeans (edamame)
		6 ounces vegetarian/soy burger
		3 ounces soy-based meat alternative
Beef / Veal		
	tripe	round steak
	fat-free all-beef hot dogs	ground beef (7% fat)
		top sirloin, fillet
		liver
		roast beef, chuck pot roast
		brisket
		flank, tenderloin
		reduced-fat hot dogs
Pork		
		pork tenderloin, ground pork
		Canadian bacon, ham
Lamb		
		lamb shank, leg, or shoulder chop
		ground lamb
Eggs		
	4 to 6 egg whites	2 whole eggs

CHOOSING NONSTARCHY VEGGIES AND FRUITS

Fill up this section of your plate with nonstarchy vegetables and fruits that give you that important vitamin C.

Your Vegetable Choices

Vegetables are foods you can eat in large amounts. They fill your stomach and fuel you with the vitamins, minerals, and fiber that you need to stay in a muscle-feeding/fat-shrinking frenzy. I categorize veggie choices by volume: The more water and fiber a vegetable has, the higher its volume. (See chart, page 63.) High-volume vegetables supply the most food with the fewest calories, so you can eat more without risking a calorie overload. Raw leafy greens like broccoli, cabbage, and salad greens are high-volume veggies, whereas parsnips, peas, and cooked beets are low volume. Keep an assortment of veggies in your freezer at all times. That way you can always add them as a quick side dish to any dinner you prepare.

If you want more food, opt for more high-volume vegetables first. This will allow you to satisfy that urge to chew without overindulging in calories. Aim to have two servings of vegetables at every meal, but don't be afraid to load up on high-volume veggies. It is hard to overeat in this category because you will fill up fast. You can mix and match. A salad can be a mixture of spring greens with a handful of diced carrots, mushrooms, celery, diced tomatoes, and sweet peppers.

Your Fruit Choices

Fruits also have a volume component, but they are listed farther down the column (starting with grapefruit) because they have higher concentrations of sugar—and thus calories. While lots of diets restrict daily fruit servings, on the Feed Muscle, Shrink Fat program you should really worry only about limiting fruits that are high in sugar. Your best bet is to find a middle ground where you eat a variety of different fruits and vegetables.

Choose freely from this list (page 63) but aim to fill up on the higher-volume fruits, such as whole apples, berries, and grapefruit, that are also higher in fiber. Any fruits with edible skins are excellent choices; think of them as vitamin C bombs wrapped with fiber. I recommend that you have two servings of fruit a day and then adjust your intake to your activity level. If, for example, you find that as you increase your activity level your hunger also goes up, you can safely add another serving or two of fruit a day. Grains are another category that you can adjust to help satisfy your body's calorie needs to keep you going.

VEGETABLES & FRUITS

These foods are listed in order from high volume to low volume. Eat more of the high-volume foods to fill you up without adding a lot of calories.

HIGH VOLUME

Raw leafy vegetables

Cooked asparagus, green beans, broccoli, red or green cabbage, cauliflower, chard, kale, sauerkraut, summer squash, zucchini

Cooked Brussels sprouts, carrots, spinach, tomato, canned mushrooms, water chestnuts, sugar snap peas; raw radishes

Cooked collards, onions, pumpkin, rutabaga, mashed acorn squash, turnips

Frozen mixed vegetables, mustard greens, parsnips, peas, cooked beets or beet greens

Grapefruit

Orange

Apple

Berries

Pineapple

Cantaloupe

Banana

Pear

Cherries

Grapes

Watermelon

Plums

Nectarine

Peach

Unsweetened applesauce

Mango

Papaya

Apricots

Prunes

Dates

LOW VOLUME

The reason I do not impose strict limits on fruits is because studies show that when you crave sugar or sweets, fruit is an excellent solution. Eating fruit is much healthier than bingeing on a high-fat, high-processed-sugar product that will sabotage your weight loss goals. When you crave a food that is more likely to feed fat cells, like a doughnut, reach for a muscle-feeding food instead, like a green apple with cottage cheese and a sprinkle of cinnamon. It is not the end of the world if you splurge on fruit. Fruit is considered a muscle-feeding friend compared with its junk food counterparts. In time you will be able to manage your consumption in this category and choose smartly among your vegetable and fruit options.

One small restriction: It should come as no surprise that sugary fruit juices are not the same as whole fruits. During this weight loss phase, you should avoid sugary fruit juices in addition to dried fruit (including raisins) and packaged dried fruit concoctions that contain added sugars.

The Vitamin C Connection

Let's return to the vitamin C component that is another key in the weight loss equation. On the Feed Muscle, Shrink Fat plan, you will consume vitamin C mostly from vegetables and fruit. The fruits and veggies with the least calories and the most vitamin C include tomatoes, salsa, grapefruit, and asparagus, which I use often in my recipes. These all have levels of vitamin C greater than your daily need, which is 75 milligrams. Salsa in particular not only adds vitamin C but is also a low-fat, low-calorie alternative to sour cream, margarine, or butter. It even counts as an extra vegetable. Although supplementing your diet with vitamin C pills can be helpful, nothing beats getting your vitamins mostly from real foods.

What else does vitamin C do? It is needed for the growth and repair of tissues in the body. It plays a role in your immunity as well as your metabolism. It is neces-

Excellent Sources of Vitamin C

blueberries	green bell peppers	raspberries
broccoli	kiwifruit	spinach
Brussels sprouts	leafy greens	strawberries
cabbage	mango	tomatoes
cantaloupe	oranges	turnip greens
cauliflower	papaya	watermelon
cranberries	pineapple	winter squash
grapefruit	potatoes	

sary to form collagen, which is used to make skin, scar tissue, tendons, ligaments, and blood vessels. It is also essential for wound healing and for the repair and maintenance of cartilage, bones, and teeth. What's more, it's a potent antioxidant.

CHOOSING WHOLE GRAINS

Let's be honest: Grain is often a code word for carbohydrates like bread, bagels, and pasta. They can be sinfully good at times and are typically the one food we find hard to restrict for long periods of time. When you deny yourself these, the tension builds and at some point you feel like you are going insane. Carbohydrates serve an essential and important function in the body, including helping you to lose weight. They help to make you feel satisfied at meals and give you sustained energy. They are also key to keeping your bowels regular and your brain fueled. If you've ever gone on a low-carb diet that restricts your intake of complex or starchy carbs for an extended period of time, you may have felt tired, weak, and brain-dead. Well, here is why: You were denying your brain and body what they want most—quick access to energy.

Kathy's Secret: As you eat more high-quality, unrefined carbs like whole grains, legumes, fruits, and vegetables, you'll find that you have less interest in eating low-quality starchy carbs like white bread and pasta, which make your insulin levels surge and your energy level drop.

Whole Grains Keep You Sane

There is a point I am making here by calling this category "whole grains." As you are aware, I am putting the focus on whole grains that offer muscle-feeding, fat-shrinking fiber. In addition to getting fiber from fruits and vegetables, you are going to obtain even more fiber from this category by switching to whole grain food varieties that can include pasta, crackers, tortillas, bread, cereal, and even cookies and some baked goods. The fiber will enhance your blood sugar stability, which in turn contributes to your feelings of fullness, satiety, and overall sense of well-being after and between meals.

Even though you will move away from refined grains like white bread and any "enriched" carbohydrate that has been stripped of its natural fiber, you will need to limit your intake in the grain category. Grains are the most calorie-dense complex carbohydrate (sugar).

Finding whole grain alternatives to your favorite breads and pastas is easy. Not only do natural food stores carry these products, but supermarket chains across the country also now stock their shelves with wholesome grains. On page 66 I have given you a list of my favorite grains and I will keep you posted on my website about new products on the market that I think you should add to your menus.

The "Grains & Starchy Vegetables" chart (page 67) displays lists from which you can choose grains that will feed your muscles and assist you in your weight loss efforts. Popular foods like white bread and regular pasta are listed as foods that you eat rarely. You would do well to transition from white ("bleached wheat flour")-flour-based products to purely whole grains and multigrains. Look for the Whole Grains Council's stamp of approval on products.

Vary Your Grain Servings
Grains occupy one category that you will need to adjust for your body type and activity level. As you start to create your own meals, limit grains to two servings a day. But if you find yourself feeling low on energy, moody, and unmotivated to work out, then by all means increase your intake of these complex carbohydrates to help keep you energized and fueled for your workouts. This will take some experimentation, but don't be afraid of trying three grain servings a day as long as you stay tuned in to how you feel. Keep a record of extra servings in your journal. If you get bloated and your weight loss seems to halt, then reduce your grains and add more protein and vegetables to your meals. Also experiment with when to add grains to your meals. You may, for instance, want a grain at lunch if you plan to work out later that afternoon.

Kathy's Favorite Grains

Brown and long grain rice	Whole/multigrain crackers
Quinoa	Wasa® high-fiber crackers
Ezekiel® breads and cereals	Kashi® multigrain crackers
Whole wheat pitas	Rye-Crisp® crackers
Kashi® cereals and oatmeal	Reduced Fat Triscuits®
Whole grain Total®	Whole wheat pasta
Product 19®	Barilla Plus® pastas
Wheaties®	Whole grain muffins
Kellogg's Bran Flakes®	Blue corn tortilla chips
McCann's Oatmeal®	Whole wheat tortillas
Granola (no added sugar)	Smart Pop® popcorn minibags
Buckwheat pancakes	Heartland® pasta

GRAINS & STARCHY VEGETABLES

Listed below are good choices for grains and starchy vegetables. They are high in fiber, so they will keep you full longer than more processed foods.

Cereals
½ cup oatmeal
¼ cup dry rolled oats
½ cup Cream of Wheat
1 cup whole grain cereal*

Breads & Tortillas
1 slice whole grain bread
1 slice rye or pumpernickel bread
½ whole wheat pita
1 whole wheat English muffin
One 6-inch corn tortilla
1 whole wheat tortilla

Rice & Pastas
½ cup brown rice
½ cup whole wheat pasta
3 tablespoons dry barley or cornmeal
¼ cup whole wheat couscous
¼ cup quinoa
⅔ cup corn grits or cooked hominy

Crackers & Chips
6 to 8 blue corn tortilla chips
5 small whole wheat or whole grain
    crackers
1 cup air-popped popcorn
½ ounce pretzels

Starchy Vegetables
½ cup cooked beans (black, pinto,
    kidney, garbanzo, etc.)
½ cup mashed butternut squash
½ cup eggplant
1 medium artichoke
⅓ cup cooked corn, lentils, split peas
1 small ear corn
1 small baked potato
2 ounces sweet potato or yam

Grains You Will Eat Rarely
1 slice white bread, including sour-
    dough and egg breads
1 small flour tortilla
½ medium bagel
1 small roll
1 small regular muffin or scone
½ ounce white flour crackers, chips,
    or pretzels
1 to 2 regular pancakes or waffles
½ cup regular pasta

(*see breakfast section, page 164)

ADD-ONS

Dessert Add-Ons

You deserve to become a bit more ambitious in this department. So when your sweet tooth strikes, here are your options:

Every-day treats. Once a day, you can still choose from the dessert list I gave you for Week 1: Fast Track 1 (page 42).

Twice-a-week recipes. You will find some of my favorite dessert recipes in the recipe section (page 236). Limit those to once a week.

Special splurges. Starting this week you can incorporate the higher-calorie treats listed below into your diet. Limit them to two times a week. These desserts will substitute for one grain at a meal during that day. For example, if you want to have three Hershey's Kisses or a slice of cake, then you'll skip having bread with dinner.

- 1 small regular cookie
- 1 small slice of cake
- 3½-ounce fat-free pudding snack
- 3 Hershey's Kisses®
- ½ cup sorbet
- ½ cup Dreyer's or Edy's Grand Light Ice Cream®
- 8 ounces fat-free frozen yogurt
- 1 slice angel food cake with berries

Dairy Add-Ons

Dairy presents a unique category close to proteins. Because dairy products contain sugar, fat, and protein, they are almost like a complete food on their own. If you are accustomed to high-fat dairy like regular cheese, whole milk, and whole yogurt, now is the time to start shifting toward leaner dairy food choices, such as low-fat and fat-free varieties. Hard cheeses are also available in several good-tasting low-fat varieties, and the experience you had in the first two weeks with my meals proved this to you.

During Weeks 3 to 6: Fat Burn, try to include two servings of dairy a day. Dairy often gets coupled with other sources of protein, as well as vegetables and fruits. For example, if you want to have an egg scramble with cheese, it is perfectly fine to adjust your protein amounts to accommodate both sources. Because cheeses and whole eggs are in the medium- to high-fat column (see chart, page 70), you will want to cut down on overall fat by either avoiding the egg yolks or selecting a reduced-fat cheese. You will also avoid using a high-fat cooking ingredient like butter and opt for a cooking spray instead.

Calcium Can Boost Weight Loss

When your body is deprived of calcium, it begins conserving it. That mechanism prompts your body to produce higher levels of the hormone calcitriol, which triggers an increased production of fat. High levels of calcitriol tell your fat cells to store themselves in the body, as well as expand. So those 40 billion fat cells you have grow bigger and fatter. You know what this means: You get bigger and fatter.

Extra calcium in your diet suppresses calcitriol, so the opposite reaction occurs: Your body breaks down more fat, and fat cells become smaller. Some studies suggest that a high-dairy diet can boost weight loss by about 70 percent. The hitch: Avoid getting your protein from high-fat sources like high-fat cheeses, yogurts, and milk. Opt for lean dairy instead. Dark leafy greens also contain calcium. You need about 1 gram (1,000 mg) of calcium a day. Women older than 50 and men older than 65 need more—about 1,500 mg a day. Most women need to take supplements to get enough calcium in their diet; my website contains more information about supplements and where to find them. Don't forget that you can opt for lactose-free milk if you are sensitive to regular milk. Vitamin D aids your body's ability to absorb calcium, which is why you find dairy products fortified with this vitamin.

My recipe section is full of ideas based on a healthy dose of dairy, from yogurt and cottage cheese selections to milk-based concoctions in my signature shakes. Several recipes call for a sprinkle of cheese. These should teach you healthy ways to include dairy in both your meals and your snacks.

DAIRY ADD-ONS

You should include two servings of dairy add-ons each day. Each item listed below is considered one serving.

Low-Fat

1 cup nonfat cottage cheese
1 cup fat-free yogurt
1 cup fat-free milk
1½ ounces whey protein powder
2 ounces low-fat cheese
1 ounce regular cheese

Medium- to High-Fat

¾ cup low-fat cottage cheese (2%)
¾ cup low-fat yogurt
¾ cup reduced-fat milk
½ cup whole milk

Fat Add-Ons

The biggest role fats have in our meals is to provide satiety and flavor. Who doesn't like a pat of butter on bread? Or a creamy dressing on a salad? Yes, there is always a time and place for butter and creamy dressing, but they can add a lot of extra calories. Use them sparingly (no more than two servings a day). There are secrets to getting the same satisfaction—and flavor—with healthier choices.

Nut butters. Nut butters like peanut, almond, and cashew contain heart-healthy monounsaturated fats. While they do contain protein, they are mostly fat (and calorie-dense) so they are placed in the fat category. Eat them instead of chips or other snack foods that are high in saturated or trans fats. Look for natural, trans-fat-free versions; avoid any that contain added sugar. You want 100 percent natural. Reduced-fat varieties also are available and may further cut your calories without cutting flavor. Just be sure to read labels and stay away from any that contain artificial ingredients or added sugar.

Whenever possible rely on olive oil or canola oil for cooking, even if you're tempted to use butter. Avoid palm oils, margarine, and anything with the words "partially hydrogenated vegetable oil."

Butter and mayonnaise. Avoid using butter and mayo, which carry lots of artery-clogging saturated fat. Steer more toward healthy fats that are rich in cholesterol-lowering monounsaturated fat. Olive oil is my favorite pick, and it should be a kitchen staple along with the less-flavorful canola oil. Remember, you will consume some saturated fat in your proteins, especially meat and cheese.

Perfect pairs. Pairing your protein with a fat is easy. The leaner the protein you choose (anything from the low-fat column in the chart on page 61), the more fat you can add to your meal. For example, if you choose high-fat salmon as your protein source, do not add a fat. Salmon is so rich in omega-3 oil that it doesn't make sense to add any fat to it. You will notice it as you fill up faster with salmon and don't feel the need for fat. But if you choose egg whites as your protein source, you may want to sprinkle some light cheese on your eggs and have a slice of toast. See? *Balance* your fat intake. Egg whites don't contain fat, so to sustain energy levels until the next meal, adding a healthy fat is smart.

Don't skip fats. Even though you are trying to shrink your fat cells, don't avoid fat. While most people could stand to reduce their dietary fat intake, it is unhealthy to completely eliminate it. Remember: Healthy fat increases the satiety value of a meal. It can help lower LDL cholesterol and elevate HDL cholesterol, help fat-soluble vitamins get around the body, and give your hair, nails, and skin a healthy glow. Also don't forget that dietary fat is not the same as body fat. Excess body fat is the combined result of a lack of exercise and overeating all nutrients.

Kathy's Secret: Instead of using fat for flavor, enliven your meals with fresh herbs, spices, or citrus. Try a bit of lemon or lime zest, garlic, ginger, mint, cilantro, horseradish, curry, or a sprinkle of vinegar!

Eat Right to Look Years Younger

Foods packed with omega-3 fatty acids have an anti-inflammatory effect on the body. Why is that so great? Well, inflammation may be the root of many evils in the body. When you cut yourself, for example, you know that inflammation—redness, swelling, pain—soon follows. Now science is telling us that inflammation may be the source of many diseases, including heart disease, stroke, and even Alzheimer's. On a smaller scale inflammation plays a role in your skin, causing blemishes, redness, swelling, and an overall bad complexion. So fight inflammation with omega-3s, which can be found in salmon, walnuts, and olive oil.

FATS & CONDIMENTS

You should limit your fat add-ons to two servings a day. Each item listed below is considered one serving.

1 tablespoon:
Oil (olive, canola, sesame, coconut, hempseed, safflower, sunflower)
Gravy (use sparingly)
Butter or mayonnaise (use sparingly)
Salad dressing (avoid any with high-fructose corn syrup)
Ground flaxseed
Nuts or seeds
2 tablespoons:
Light salad dressing
Light gravy
Light cream cheese
Light sour cream
Low-fat guacamole
Cholesterol-lowering spread (Smart Balance®, Take Control®)
Light mayonnaise
Barbecue sauce, teriyaki sauce, ketchup (avoid those with high-fructose corn syrup)
Nut butters (peanut, almond, cashew, etc.)
Other amounts:
¼ avocado
½ cup salsa, tomato juice, or tomato sauce
10 olives, any color
1 teaspoon all-natural sugar or agave nectar (See page 44 for notes and guidelines on sugar.)
Freebies
lemon juice, lime juice, mustard, light soy sauce, vinegar, cooking spray (olive- or canola-oil based), spices, fresh herbs, salt & ground pepper

ADJUST PORTION SIZES TO SUIT YOUR NEEDS

I have built in plenty of flexibility to help you tailor this program to your needs. Not everyone enjoys three meals a day, so you will find ideas for breaking up your calorie load to create mini meals and snacks scattered throughout the day.

If my daily meal plan feels like too much food for you, then you shouldn't feel pressured to eat more than you need. Conversely if you don't feel like you're eating enough food, I will show you how to make needed adjustments. You should not have to count calories and grams or measure foods on a kitchen scale. I want you to become so attuned to your body's needs, including its level of hunger and sense of fullness, that you can decide for yourself the proper portions for you. Not only is everyone's body different, but everyone's level of activity is different. One day you may be high on the activity scale, and the next you may be mostly sitting in front of a computer and not moving much. Because activity levels change constantly, there is no magic calorie total that will meet your individual and perpetually evolving needs. Calorie consumption should be viewed more broadly. One day you may be hungrier and actually need more calories than the next. Don't be afraid to respond to that true hunger and take in an extra 100 to 200 calories.

You are training your body to feel satisfied with the right amount of calories *for you*. My hope is that you can do away with "rules" once you finish my program so you can successfully adopt this way of eating as a lifetime practice. I understand that the learning curve for shifting your way of eating can feel restrictive. It is human nature to resist change. But with the right attitude toward all that awaits you once you become a healthier person, the benefits outweigh the frustrations.

Increase Proteins and Vegetables/Fruits First

Every meal starts with a protein and a healthy serving of high-volume produce. Then you can add a grain and dairy twice a day. As you sense the need to give your calorie consumption a boost to meet your activity level, start by increasing protein and vegetable/fruit portions, then add more grains and dairy if you still don't feel like you are eating enough fuel to satisfy your energy needs. It is much easier to reach your satiety level through protein and fibrous vegetables/fruits than through dairy and grains that have simple sugars that easily rush into the bloodstream.

Track Hunger with Your Journal

The key to knowing where and when to increase foods is to listen to your hunger. If you undereat eventually you will overeat. Use your journal to track hunger and level of satiety after each meal. As you lose body fat and increase muscle mass, you are retraining how many calories your body needs to run efficiently. You are maximizing your immune system and cardiovascular capacity in the meantime.

But I'm Still Hungry!

If you find yourself still hungry after a meal, and you thought you chose the right portions using my guidelines, here are some explanations:

Your body hasn't registered that it is full. It takes your stomach about 20 minutes to feel satiated, so wait at least that long before eating seconds. If you wait and still want more, have a few more ounces of lean protein or high-fiber vegetables.

You ate too quickly. Try chewing your food slowly and deliberately, putting your knife and fork down after every bite. This way you will enjoy your meals more and need less to be satisfied. Have a conversation or read a book to slow yourself down.

You are dehydrated. Many people mistake thirst for hunger, so before a meal or snack, drink an 8-ounce glass of water, wait 10 minutes, and see if your hunger abates.

You are shortchanging one of your food groups. Usually it is protein, so try increasing the amount you eat by a few ounces to see if that helps. You also can consume more raw or steamed vegetables to make you feel satisfied longer.

You are premenstrual—craving fat and sugar. Hormone levels affect hunger, so during that time be particularly conscious of your eating habits and portion sizes. Take extra care to select healthy treats that will level off your cravings.

You are skipping meals. Remember to follow the three- to four-hour guideline.

LIVING LEAN SUMMARY

Instead of thinking in terms of what not to eat, think of what you can eat. Below is a list of heart-smart alternatives that allow you to have the foods you love without the unhealthy fats or refined carbs.

Instead of this ...	... Eat this
Poultry with skin	Poultry without skin
Full-fat dairy products	Reduced-fat and fat-free dairy products
Plain pasta	Whole wheat, quinoa, or fiber-rich pasta
Butter or margarine	Vegetable oil, olive oil or soft, trans-fat–free margarine
Eggs	Some whole eggs (Omega and organic varieties are best) mixed with egg whites or egg substitute
Regular versions of snack foods	Baked and trans-fat-free versions of chips, crackers, and other favorites
Low-fiber breakfast cereal	High-fiber breakfast cereal
Refined bread, English muffins, and pita	Whole grain and fiber-rich bread products
Protein bars	Fiber-rich cereal bars

ASK KATHY: COMMON QUESTIONS

Do you still have questions about the Feed Muscle, Shrink Fat Diet? These are some of the things people ask me about most.

Q. ■ How can I get more fiber in my diet?

A. ■ Try to get at least 25 to 30 grams of fiber each day. Fiber helps with feeling satisfied after a meal and helps maintain regularity. When it comes to fiber, here are the best foods to eat:

Blackberries	Blueberries	Apples
Asparagus	Green beans	Beets
Broccoli	Corn	Peas*
Black beans*	Pinto beans*	Lima beans*
Lentils*	Oat bran*	Barley*
Citrus fruits*	Flaxseed* (sprinkle on cereal or add to shakes)	

Good sources of soluble fiber, the heart-healthy kind

Q. ■ My weight loss has slowed down. What can I do?

A. ■ Hitting a plateau is a natural part of weight loss. The good news is that this could be a sign that your body has become more fit and efficient—using less energy to get more done. It also could be a sign of an invisible transition taking place inside the body whereby you're still losing actual fat, but weightwise that loss is hiding behind some water retention and gains in muscle mass. This is when patience is in order.

If you don't see the scale tick downward again in a week, it may be time to reflect on your exercise and diet habits. Sometimes pushing past a plateau and continuing to see results means increasing the intensity of your workouts and pushing your body harder. Keeping the body guessing doesn't let it get used to your workouts and is what keeps you moving forward. On the diet front check your choices and make sure you haven't been veering too far from the guidelines.

Q. ■ What can I do about late-night hunger?

A. ■ If you're encountering late-night hunger, first take a look at what you're eating for dinner and make sure you're eating enough to feel balanced and satisfied. If you had a satisfying and balanced meal but you still really want a little something to eat, it's always best to eat some protein. A few almonds or slices of turkey are good choices. If that's not enough, add a vegetable or piece of fruit to the protein. Watch your portions, but know that if you're hungry, protein and produce are the best things to reach for.

Q. ■ Can I have an occasional cocktail?

A. ■ Did you know that a piña colada has 640 calories, which is more than a Big Mac? Here are some other alarming cocktail calorie counts that will get you thinking twice next time you place your order:

Long Island iced tea: 780 calories
Margarita: 740 calories
White Russian: 425 calories
Mai tai: 350 calories
Gin/Vodka tonic: 200 calories
Cosmopolitan: 150 calories

Q. ■ Are there any banned foods on this diet?

A. ■ I want you to make this important shift in your mindset: Forget about banning or limiting specific food groups. Instead focus on which nutrients are going to support your health and weight loss goals. In other words, if you've been counting carbohydrates or fat grams, it's time to develop a new perspective. With the Feed Muscle, Shrink Fat plan, carbohydrates and fats will still be part of the language, but turning the attention to the three metabolism-maximizing nutrients can revolutionize your weight loss experience. It will take a lot of the confusion out of deciding what to eat.

Q. ■ **I don't like lifting weights. I worry that I'll get too bulky if I even try. Why is it so important?**

A. ■ Weight training is not only for jocks and muscleheads. It's vital to our ability to stay looking and feeling our best because it helps build and preserve lean muscle mass. We begin to lose muscle mass naturally at about the age of 30, so maintaining as much as we can becomes critical. Cardio is invaluable to any fitness program, but too many people get caught up counting calories on the treadmill and disregard strength training completely.

It's very difficult to build lean muscle mass and bone density through cardio alone; moreover, strength training is the ticket to boosting your metabolism—providing up to a 15 percent increase in metabolic rate. Cardio itself will burn calories and kick your metabolism up a notch, but without more muscle mass to demand a higher metabolism, you'll still be working in a low gear. Strength training also keeps your metabolism humming longer after a workout than cardio alone would. In fact too much cardio can put pressure on your adrenal glands, leading to fatigue and stress on your body that will work against your weight loss goals. You shouldn't worry about getting bulky; lifting weights doesn't mean adding bulk to your body.

My Matrix system will sculpt and define your muscles while at the same time burning fat. It will also help prevent injury, minimize the loss of bone mass, and even release endorphins to improve your sense of well-being. Finally it's worth noting that strength training has been shown over and over again to reduce the signs and symptoms of numerous diseases and chronic conditions, including arthritis, diabetes, osteoporosis, obesity, back pain, and depression. With so many potential benefits, how can you say no? Strength training is the ultimate way to slow down your physiological clock.

LIVING LEAN SHOPPING LIST

Take the guesswork out of your grocery shopping by keeping the formula in mind: pro-tein + vitamin C + fiber. This will lead you to choose lean proteins, high-fiber fruits and vegetables packed with vitamin C, and whole grains. Then think about what ingredients you need to create your snacks for the week and decide which dairy and fats you want to add. You can break down your shopping list this way too.

Proteins	Fruits/Vegetables	Grains
skinless chicken breasts	apples, oranges	7-grain bread
salmon steaks	bag of frozen berries	steel-cut oatmeal
turkey slices (deli)	asparagus	brown rice
fish of the day	spinach, broccoli	
lean ground beef	bell peppers	
	mixed greens	

Dairy and Fat (Add-ons)	Other Ingredients for Snacks and Shakes	
olive oil	hummus	
sour cream	nuts	
low-fat cheese	whole grain crackers	
3 fat-free yogurts	vanilla protein powder	
peanut butter		
fat-free milk		

LIVING LEAN SHOPPING LIST

Take the guesswork out of your grocery shopping by keeping the formula in mind: protein + vitamin C + fiber. This will lead you to choose lean proteins, high-fiber fruits and vegetables packed with vitamin C, and whole grains. Then think about what ingredients you need to create your snacks for the week and decide which dairy and fats you want to add. You can break down your shopping list this way too.

Proteins	Fruits/Vegetables	Grains
Dairy and Fat (Add-ons)	**Other Ingredients for Snacks and Shakes**	

LIVING LEAN JOURNAL

Keeping a journal is so important to success. It tells you a lot about your eating habits. See the sample below, then turn the page for your own blank journal page.

Day: **Short-term weekly goal:**

Date: / / **Daily goal:**

Meal	Hunger level before eating	Hunger level after eating	
Breakfast	Starving ☒ Normal ☐ Stuffed ☐	Starving ☐ Normal ☒ Stuffed ☐	Protein: *egg white omelet* Fruits/Vegetable (vit. C): *the omelet had spinach and tomatoes in it* Grain (Fiber): *1 slice of whole grain toast, plain*
Lunch	Starving ☒ Normal ☐ Stuffed ☐	Starving ☐ Normal ☐ Stuffed ☒	Protein: *grilled chicken sandwich from a restaurant (ate with coworkers)* Fruits/Vegetable (vit. C): *the sandwich had lettuce and tomato on it* Grain (Fiber): *bun (but wasn't whole wheat)*
Dinner	Starving ☐ Normal ☒ Stuffed ☐	Starving ☐ Normal ☒ Stuffed ☐	Protein: *deli turkey breast (in my salad)* Fruits/Vegetable (vit. C): *big salad with lettuce, tomatoes, cucumbers, and peppers* Grain (Fiber): *whole grain crackers*
Snacks	Starving ☐ Normal ☒ Stuffed ☐	Starving ☐ Normal ☒ Stuffed ☐	*cucumber boats* *yogurt with berries*
Water	☒ ☒ ☒ ☒ ☐ ☐ ☐ ☐ ☐ ☐		
Exercise	Workouts Completed: *Matrix Workout + Walking 2 miles* My Intensitiy Level Was: ☐ High ☒ Moderate ☐ Low ☐ Very Low		

Today's Experiences: *I didn't do so well at lunch. Friends at work invited me out to lunch at a diner and there wasn't much healthy food to eat. But I do feel good about eating well at breakfast and dinner. Plus I had a great workout!*

LIVING LEAN JOURNAL

Make copies of this blank journal page and fill it in each day. Every week look back and note changes you could make to have even greater success the following week.

Day: _____ **Short-term weekly goal:** _____

Date: / / **Daily goal:** _____

Meal	Hunger level before eating	Hunger level after eating	
Breakfast	Starving ☐ Normal ☐ Stuffed ☐	Starving ☐ Normal ☐ Stuffed ☐	Protein: _____ Fruits/Vegetable (vit. C): _____ Grain (Fiber): _____
Lunch	Starving ☐ Normal ☐ Stuffed ☐	Starving ☐ Normal ☐ Stuffed ☐	Protein: _____ Fruits/Vegetable (vit. C): _____ Grain (Fiber): _____
Dinner	Starving ☐ Normal ☐ Stuffed ☐	Starving ☐ Normal ☐ Stuffed ☐	Protein: _____ Fruits/Vegetable (vit. C): _____ Grain (Fiber): _____
Snacks	Starving ☐ Normal ☐ Stuffed ☐	Starving ☐ Normal ☐ Stuffed ☐	_____ _____
Water			
Exercise	Workouts Completed: _____ My Intensitiy Level Was: ☐ High ☐ Moderate ☐ Low ☐ Very Low		

Today's Experiences: _____
_____
_____

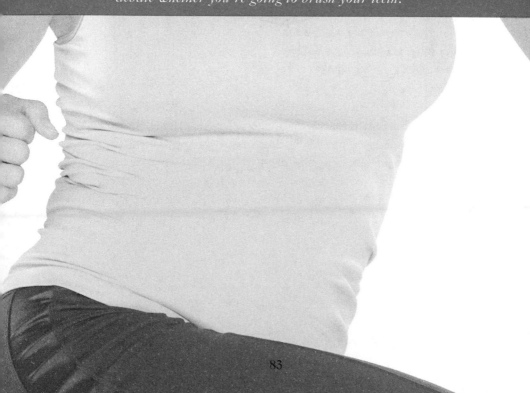

PART 2: THE WORKOUT

Exercise is nonnegotiable, just like brushing your teeth. And you don't debate whether you're going to brush your teeth.

People often ask me what is the most helpful lesson I've learned about staying in shape, and I tell them this: Exercise is as significant as what I eat. It lifts my spirits and attitude, making me feel so much younger than my age. It gets me going in the morning, keeps me focused, and takes the edge off if I'm stressed and tense. Exercise makes me physically stronger and toned, which is nearly impossible to achieve just through diet. I've also learned that staying in shape is much easier than getting in shape.

Like all great exercise programs, my Feed Muscle, Shrink Fat plan will accelerate your metabolism and burn calories. But my program also incorporates one of the best-kept secrets to successful weight loss and healthy living: strength training. Strength training builds and preserves lean muscle tissue and helps shrink fat. In Part 1 you learned how "feeding" muscle helps you become a leaner, fitter person by keeping your metabolism humming and your energy level high. In addition to diet, exercise is an essential component to feeding your muscles and, of course, shrinking fat.

In Week 1 and Week 2, you start with 10-minute workouts—10 simple exercises a day that take just one minute each to complete. All the moves are based on my revolutionary Matrix exercise system, which you will learn about shortly. They offer an efficient, total body workout in little time. Here is how your workouts will break down:

Upper-body exercises: 2 days a week
Lower-body exercises: 2 days a week
Core exercises: 2 days a week
Rest: 1 day a week

You will be amazed by what you can accomplish in just 10 minutes, strengthening your heart and lungs while building lean muscle mass and transforming your body's ratio of fat to muscle. In other words you will shift the balance of power from your fat cells to your muscle cells. When you combine this exercise plan with the super nutrition in the Feed Muscle, Shrink Fat Diet, your body will have no reason to retain extra fat, and you will get maximum results in just six weeks.

THE MATRIX WORKOUT OVERVIEW

After the age of 30, we all lose ¼ pound of muscle mass each year if we aren't strength training. With less muscle our metabolism slows and we are more likely to gain fat. Remember, while muscle is metabolically active (each pound of muscle can burn 35 to 50 calories a day), stored fat is not active, so it burns far fewer calories. The more muscle you have, the more calories you burn 24/7, regardless of what you are doing.

To understand why my Feed Muscle, Shrink Fat Workout is so successful, let's talk about the differences between strength (or weight) training and aerobic exercise. Both types of exercise burn calories and build muscle mass but at very different rates.

• **Aerobic exercise**, which refers mainly to cardio work that raises your heart rate for an extended period, burns fat and glucose *during* exercise.

• **Strength (or weight) training** utilizes fat and glucose for hours (and sometimes days) *after* exercising, so your metabolism stays slightly elevated for a longer period of time following a strength training session than after an aerobic workout. This is called the afterburn, which is fueled mostly by fat cells. Your body is working hard to reoxygenate your blood and restore circulatory hormones. This state of elevated oxygen use means a state of elevated calorie burning. How long the afterburn lasts can vary from a few hours to days, depending on the type of exercise you choose, its intensity, and how your body responds to the exercise.

THE IDEAL WORKOUT

Your optimal workout, then, should include both strength and cardio training—which is exactly what you will get on my Feed Muscle, Shrink Fat program.

The Matrix: Strength Training

With my patented Matrix strength training program, you will work your whole body, including upper, lower, and core. You can emphasize a particular area for maximum results as other areas fully recover. The combination of moves you'll do in my Matrix workout will progress over the weeks and become incrementally more rigorous. As you build your strength and endurance, and as your body gets comfortable with the moves, you will add new challenges by increasing duration, weight, and speed.

Cardio Workouts for Aerobic Exercise

To realize aerobic benefits in your workouts, starting in Week 3 you will add 10-minute cardio workouts into your exercise routines (starting on page 98). You can also do burst training, which is alternating spurts of low- and high-intensity cardio. Think of leisurely jogging (low intensity) versus flat-out running (high intensity). Cardio burst training can be done in any aerobic activity, including cycling, running, and swimming. You simply turn up the heat for a short period of time and go a little harder.

Burst training has numerous benefits, from maximizing fat burn after your workout to increasing hormones such as human growth hormone, that facilitate fat loss. It adds variety to your workouts so you stay motivated and enthusiastic. It fosters a stronger cardiovascular fitness level and taps fat stores. In fact cardio burst training is a fat burner in itself. Research shows that during a cardio burst workout, fat-burning enzymes in the muscles increase to a much greater extent than during other types of workouts. And burst training may be the only way to break down intramuscular fat (fat located inside muscle tissue) into its fatty-acid components so it can then be used as energy and burned off.

Advance at Your Own Pace

I designed the Feed Muscle, Shrink Fat Workout program to suit all fitness levels.

Basic Level. You can stick with the 10-minute baseline workout from Weeks 1 and 2 for as long as you need.

Intermediate Level. Follow the entire workout as outlined.

Advanced Level. When you are ready for additional physical challenges, refer to the advanced six-week Matrix program, which will accelerate the progression of the workout—and its resulting payoffs—starting in Week 2.

UNDERSTANDING THE MATRIX WORKOUT

"Matrix" is the name for my innovative system of exercise moves that employ a three-dimensional space. By performing a series of fluid motions in all directions—such as forward/back, side to side, and rotational—you simultaneously engage multiple muscles, along with joints, ligaments, and tendons, so that your body works as a unit. The Matrix is one of the most efficient ways to tone the body quickly and completely. It brings back definition to waistlines, sculpts arms and legs, lifts butts, tightens thighs, and more. It is an incredibly powerful method of physical conditioning that results in a body that is longer, leaner, lighter, and most important, able to handle the physical rigors of everyday life.

The Matrix is based on functional training, which was developed by world-renowned physical therapists and professionals who specialize in high-performance exercise physiology and kinesiology. Instead of training one muscle at a time, which used to be the fashion, the Matrix follows the "integration" method of physical training. For example, one Matrix move is called the Chop, and it entails bending, twisting, lifting, reaching, squatting, lunging, and extending, all in one sequence of integrated movements.

It is not that there is anything wrong with isolating muscles and training them as you would in, say, a bicep curl. But there are limitations with that kind of training. You are not getting the improved function, balance, flexibility, and coordination that come only when you treat the body like an integrated whole. By contrast integrated movement is natural movement. In daily life muscles work together. When you get on an airplane, for example, you must bend, twist, and stretch in the narrow aisle to hoist your luggage and place it overhead. That twisting, bending, and placing is an example of the compound, integrated movements that occur every day at the grocery store, when taking out the trash, or when putting the kids in the car. The Matrix is a holistic style of training that ultimately protects you against the aches, pains, and risk of injury that accompany age. Moreover because it draws upon how we move naturally in everyday life, it gives the body what it needs to respond more quickly to signals from the brain, optimize coordination and balance, and gain maximum agility.

The Core Difference

You can't perform these movements easily, effectively, and safely unless you have built a strong core of supporting muscles, using exercises that mimic daily demands. That is where my core Matrix exercises come in. And there is a great side benefit: All the bracing and stabilizing at the core creates the most toned stomach and midsection you can get. You will even be working those "forgotten" muscles that lend a hand to your back, underarms, thighs, and belly—some of the hardest areas to work.

Adding Weights

The Matrix uses your own body's weight as resistance. But when you are ready to challenge yourself further, try using the extra weights that are optional in many of the moves. By adding more weight you push your metabolism higher, increase the demands on your muscles so they burn more energy and build more lean mass, and up your body's oxygen use for the best calorie burning.

You decide how much weight to add. You can buy free weights directly from my website or at your local sporting goods store. Choose weights that are comfortable to grip. A good starter set includes 3-, 5-, and 8-pound weights.

Using a Body Ball

While all of the exercises can be done on the floor, you also may perform the exercises using a body ball, which is available on my website. Also called stability balls, these were invented by the Swiss to help people with injuries rehabilitate their arms and legs. But they were quickly adopted by the fitness world for their versatility and adaptability. A 55-cm ball is appropriate for people 4'11" to 5'5" tall; a 65-cm is for people 5'6" to 5'11" tall. Using a ball will intensify your workout. Wherever you find a reference to the ball during the exercises, know that you can skip it and perform the exercises on the floor.

CONSISTENCY IS KEY

For more than 25 years I have exercised every day. Now does that mean I do full, hour-long workouts every day? No. Some days I may be able to fit in only 10 minutes or 30 minutes of exercise. Other days I have time for a strenuous, two-hour hike. But whether it is 10 minutes or 60, I make sure I work out. Not only because I want to burn off last night's dinner and because I know it will improve my overall health, but because I don't want to fall out of practice. That's what I mean by consistency. If you fall out of the habit, simply get right back on track.

VARIETY ADDS INTEREST

Some people get in an exercise rut by making the mistake of always doing the same workout at the same place at the same time of day for the same amount of time. The body adapts and plateaus, and frustration sets in. This is a setup for losing momentum and interest because one day off becomes 10 or more. Mixing up speed, intensity, and type of exercise is key to getting results. The Feed Muscle, Shrink Fat Workout plan is designed with enough variety to avoid these ruts.

Mix Up Your Routine for a Change of Pace

Remember, it all adds up. Exercise is cumulative. It doesn't have to be done in a 20-, 30-, or 60-minute session. Split up your workouts if you like. Do a 10-minute Matrix routine in the morning and another 10 minutes later that day combined with an additional aerobic activity, such as a long walk after dinner. At the start of this program, you will do the 10-minute Matrix exercises, but I hope you build longer workouts as the weeks progress. Feel free to be creative with the order of the routines, especially after the structured six-week plan. The beauty of the Matrix is that it opens the door for so much variety and customization. I designed these six weeks so they gradually become more intense, but you are ultimately in charge.

Adjust the Intensity
There are four main ways to increase or decrease the intensity of your workouts for something different.

1. Weight. I give you the option to add weights, but you can choose how much weight to add, if any.

2. Speed. I give you a recommended number of exercise repetitions, which is typically 15 to 30 repetitions per minute, depending on the particular move. You can choose to slow it down and do fewer repetitions per minute.

3. Range of motion. Because you squat, lunge, reach, bend, and twist, you can start by going through a minimal range of motion and then gradually go for greater depth and reach.

4. Duration. In Week 3 the program calls for 20 minutes in the Matrix, combining more moves and spending more time working out. Don't feel pressured to do the full 20 minutes if you are not ready. You can stay at the level of Weeks 1 and 2 for as long as you like until you feel ready to step it up.

FIND YOUR OWN PACE

When you are starting to learn my Matrix exercises, it is critical that you focus on form and progress slowly. It is important not only that the muscles have a chance to be stimulated and strengthen but also that the connective tissues surrounding the muscles strengthen. These functional Matrix exercises have more than one skill involved to perform each properly. For example, Squat with Side Lift and Overhead Press has three skills. All three skills have form points that need to be learned. As you perform the exercises, continually do form checks, particularly of your posture

Write It Down
Use your journal to record which exercises you do, plus their duration and intensity. This will help you pinpoint where you are doing well—and where you need to improve. For instance, maybe you are consistent with your Matrix workouts but are not challenging yourself. Watch your journal for clues.

Bust Those Exercise Excuses!

It is not always easy to find the motivation to work out. Even I have my days when I want to skip exercising. I can be tired, cranky, overwhelmed with other things to do, and simply not in the mood. So what do I do? A few things:

✳ I think about how I will feel after my workout. Once I get moving, the blood will start circulating and my outlook will change in a flash. Then the endorphins will kick in and I will feel clear-minded, energized, and alive.

✳ I consider the social aspect of a workout with friends, family, and even my staff and business colleagues. For example, I will spend an afternoon on a hike with my daughters, join a friend at her favorite Spinning or yoga class, or use my fitness time for brainstorming and connecting with my staff. If I can include others in my workout plans, it's harder to back out.

✳ I approach the workout as a challenge instead of a chore to check off. I use the workout as way to learn more about my body, explore its limits, and flush out my emotions.

✳ I listen to my body and don't force it to do what it resists. If I don't feel like adding speed work to my workout today, I don't. Simple as that!

and the activity in your core, so your body memorizes good form and technique and starts to be aware of the core's activity.

Everyone is at a different fitness level, and this program is designed for all levels. I typically refer to three categories of people:

1. Just starting out: This is someone who hasn't exercised in the last year or who is returning after a break.

2. Exercises a little: This person is more active but isn't consistent with her workouts.

3. Exercises regularly: This person has already developed the discipline to stick with a program.

You have to be the judge of your body. My wish is that you continually challenge yourself and set new standards as you move ahead. If you do this, instead of hitting a plateau your fitness level will continue to increase, gradually allowing you to burn more and more calories in less time.

If you feel that your body hasn't recuperated enough since your last workout, pace yourself by modifying the next session and perhaps lowering the intensity. You can do this simply by taking the tempo down or lowering the amount of weight you add. It is important to give your body the recovery time it needs. Find a balance between pushing forward and pulling back to recover. My workout program is designed with recovery in mind. You will not focus on the same muscles day after day. You will also find a collection of 12 stretches to do after your workout to help cool down the body and support its recovery.

THE IMPORTANCE OF THE WARM-UP

Warming up is an essential part of exercise, so never skip it. During your warm-up more blood travels to the working muscles, which prepares your body for the workout ahead. By gradually raising your heart rate and increasing your body temperature, it actually makes the workout more efficient. Starting out too quickly can cause lactic acid to build up. Lactic acid creates that burning feeling in your muscles, which can interfere with your overall workout if you need to recover. Warm muscles stretch more easily so you are less likely to injure them.

On the Matrix, every first move you do is a warm-up. But we all need a different amount of time to get into gear. So if you need to, do the first move a little longer or try another rhythmic move until your body feels ready to go on.

DEALING WITH PLATEAUS

Plateaus are not stumbling blocks. They are a natural part of life, and everyone, from elite athletes to beginners, experiences them. Still, while sitting on a plateau you may feel stuck and think you have had enough.

Not so fast! There is good news in plateaus. They happen because your body has become more efficient. It is more capable of handling the same routine. It doesn't have to work as hard to get the workout done. Your muscles are trained, and the most important muscle of all—your heart—is up to speed by pumping more blood with less effort. These are all signs that you are a more fit person. But now you need to keep the body challenged. When it is not challenged anymore, it stays at the same level.

Remember that you are in charge of the progression of the workout. You can

Kathy's Secret: Reminder: In the beginning it is most important to work on form and technique. If you have time to cover only half of the exercises recommended for the day, that is still a great investment in your future health.

91

take it to greater lenghts by using heavier weights, going more quickly, changing the order of the exercise moves, or doubling up the duration of the workout.
As soon as you sense that your body is becoming used to a workout, think about
taking it up a notch to surprise your body. Your workouts may be too easy if you
don't feel any muscle soreness the next day following a "tough" workout.

Plateaus also can be psychological. However, given my program's variety, you
are not likely to experience this kind of plateau in these six weeks.

MOVING BEYOND WEEK 7

Once you reach Week 7, you plan your own workouts based on the strong foundation you have built during Weeks 1 through 6. You have many options. You can
continue to mix Matrix routines with the cardio work of your choice. You can
do the Matrix moves in the sequences used during the past six weeks or mix and
match exercises to keep your workout fresh and varied.

Consistency remains important. If you are short on time and can do only a
10-minute workout, use a workout from Week 1. Don't drop the entire workout
because of time constraints. Results are completely dependent on consistency.

These moves can go anywhere and be integrated into other activities. They can be
done in a hotel room, on a beach while on vacation, or at the office. They are powerful tools that you can use for years and years to stay in the best shape of your life.

The Fat-Burning Walk Option

I am a big proponent of walking because it is cheap and simple. I have created numerous walking programs, which you can find on my website. Adding a walk to your exercise regimen can magnify your results. You can easily
mix up and shift the intensity of a walk by changing your speed, going longer
distances, and finding grades that take you uphill or downhill. You can even
get the benefits of cardio burst training by including intervals in your walks—
short, brief bursts of walking as fast as you can. For accelerated results in
Weeks 1 and 2, add a 20-minute walk to your 10-minute Matrix routines.
In the following weeks try to add 5 to 10 minutes more each week to your
walk. Walking also can serve as a great warm-up when you do it before your
Matrix workout.

THE MATRIX WORKOUT: WEEKS 1–6

The following is a summary of the Matrix workout. The workout progresses starting in the third week and builds up to a 30-minute session.

WEEK 1: 10 MINUTES PER DAY

DAY 1: Upper-Body Workout

DAY 2: Lower-Body Workout

DAY 3: Core Workout

DAY 4: Upper-Body Workout

DAY 5: Lower-Body Workout

DAY 6: Core Workout

DAY 7: REST

WEEK 2: 10 MINUTES PER DAY

DAY 1: Lower-Body Workout

DAY 2: Upper-Body Workout

DAY 3: Core Workout

DAY 4: Lower-Body Workout

DAY 5: Upper-Body Workout

DAY 6: Core Workout

DAY 7: REST

WEEK 3: 20 MINUTES PER DAY

DAY 1: Upper-Body Workout 10 minutes + Core Workout 10 minutes

DAY 2: Lower-Body Workout 10 minutes + Cardio Workout 10 minutes

DAY 3: Upper-Body Workout 10 minutes + Core Workout 10 minutes

DAY 4: Lower-Body Workout 10 minutes + Cardio Workout 10 minutes

DAY 5: Upper-Body Workout 10 minutes + Core Workout 10 minutes

DAY 6: Lower-Body Workout 10 minutes + Cardio Workout 10 minutes

DAY 7: REST

WEEK 4: 20 MINUTES PER DAY*
DAY 1: Lower-Body Workout 10 minutes + Cardio Workout 10 minutes
DAY 2: Upper-Body Workout 10 minutes + Core Workout 10 minutes
DAY 3: Lower-Body Workout 10 minutes + Cardio Workout 10 minutes
DAY 4: Upper-Body Workout 10 minutes + Core Workout 10 minutes
DAY 5: Lower-Body Workout 10 minutes + Cardio Workout 10 minutes
DAY 6: Upper-Body Workout 10 minutes + Core Workout 10 minutes
DAY 7: REST

WEEK 5: 20 MINUTES PER DAY
DAY 1: Upper-Body Workout 10 minutes + Cardio Workout 10 minutes
DAY 2: Lower-Body Workout 10 minutes + Core Workout 10 minutes
DAY 3: Upper-Body Workout 10 minutes + Cardio Workout 10 minutes
DAY 4: Lower-Body Workout 10 minutes + Core Workout 10 minutes
DAY 5: Upper-Body Workout 10 minutes + Cardio Workout 10 minutes
DAY 6: Lower-Body Workout 10 minutes + Core Workout 10 minutes
DAY 7: REST

WEEK 6: 20 MINUTES PER DAY
DAY 1: Lower-Body Workout 10 minutes + Core Workout 10 minutes
DAY 2: Upper-Body Workout 10 minutes + Cardio Workout 10 minutes
DAY 3: Lower-Body Workout 10 minutes + Core Workout 10 minutes
DAY 4: Upper-Body Workout 10 minutes + Cardio Workout 10 minutes
DAY 5: Lower-Body Workout 10 minutes + Core Workout 10 minutes
DAY 6: Upper-Body Workout 10 minutes + Cardio Workout 10 minutes
DAY 7: REST

By Week 4 your body acclimates to the exercises well, and you will be able to perform them with good form and technique. This is when you may choose to add more intensity and really focus on form. Consider using a slightly heavier weight or doing a second set of moves (10 more minutes).

THE ADVANCED MATRIX WORKOUT

The following is an advanced version of the Matrix workout. It accelerates the progression starting in the second week and builds up to a 30-minute workout. This also provides of good example of how you can mix and match workouts to keep the program varied and intense.

WEEK 1: 10 MINUTES PER DAY
DAY 1: Upper-Body Workout
DAY 2: Lower-Body Workout
DAY 3: Core Workout
DAY 4: Upper-Body Workout
DAY 5: Lower-Body Workout
DAY 6: Core Workout
DAY 7: REST

WEEK 2: 20 MINUTES PER DAY
DAY 1: Upper-Body Workout 10 minutes + Core Workout 10 minutes
DAY 2: Lower-Body Workout 10 minutes + Cardio Workout 10 minutes
DAY 3: Upper-Body Workout 10 minutes + Core Workout 10 minutes
DAY 4: Lower-Body Workout 10 minutes + Cardio Workout 10 minutes
DAY 5: Upper-Body Workout 10 minutes + Core Workout 10 minutes
DAY 6: Lower-Body Workout 10 minutes + Cardio Workout 10 minutes
DAY 7: REST

WEEK 3: 20 MINUTES PER DAY
DAY 1: Upper-Body Workout 10 minutes + Cardio Workout 10 minutes
DAY 2: Lower-Body Workout 10 minutes + Core Workout 10 minutes
DAY 3: Upper-Body Workout 10 minutes + Cardio Workout 10 minutes
DAY 4: Lower-Body Workout 10 minutes + Core Workout 10 minutes
DAY 5: Upper-Body Workout 10 minutes + Cardio Workout 10 minutes
DAY 6: Lower-Body Workout 10 minutes + Core Workout 10 minutes
DAY 7: REST

WEEK 4: 30 MINUTES PER DAY*
DAY 1: Upper-Body Workout 10 minutes + Core Workout 10 minutes + Second Set of Upper Body Workout 10 minutes
DAY 2: Lower-Body Workout 10 minutes + Cardio Workout 10 minutes + Second Set of Lower Body Workout 10 minutes
DAY 3: Upper-Body Workout 10 minutes + Core Workout 10 minutes + Second Set of Upper Body Workout 10 minutes
DAY 4: Lower-Body Workout 10 minutes + Cardio Workout 10 minutes + Second Set of Lower Body Workout 10 minutes
DAY 5: Upper-Body Workout 10 minutes + Core Workout 10 minutes + Second Set of Upper Body Workout 10 minutes
DAY 6: Lower-Body Workout 10 minutes + Cardio Workout 10 minutes + Second Set of Lower Body Workout 10 minutes
DAY 7: REST

WEEK 5: 30 MINUTES PER DAY*
DAY 1: Lower-Body Workout 10 minutes + Core Workout 10 minutes + Second Set of Lower Body Workout 10 minutes
DAY 2: Upper-Body Workout 10 minutes + Cardio Workout 10 minutes + Second Set of Upper Body Workout 10 minutes
DAY 3: Lower-Body Workout 10 minutes + Core Workout 10 minutes + Second Set of Lower Body Workout 10 minutes
DAY 4: Upper-Body Workout 10 minutes + Cardio Workout 10 minutes + Second Set of Upper Body Workout 10 minutes
DAY 5: Lower-Body Workout 10 minutes + Core Workout 10 minutes + Second Set of Lower Body Workout 10 minutes
DAY 6: Upper-Body Workout 10 minutes + Cardio Workout 10 minutes + Second Set of Upper Body Workout 10 minutes
DAY 7: REST

By Week 4 your body will get used to doing the exercises and you will be able to perform them with good form and technique. You may be able to use a slightly heavier weight in the second set. Listen to your body. Additionally in Weeks 4 and 5, another option for organizing the workouts is to do the entire upper-body workout, repeat the entire upper-body workout, then do the cardio or core workout rather than sandwich the cardio or core workout between the two sets of upper-body workouts. It is not efficient to do one exercise, repeat it, then move on to the next exercise. For example, if you do Side Lateral Lifts with Balance, your shoulders will be fatigued. To do another set you need rest, particularly for your shoulders. It is not time-efficient to wait for your shoulders to rest, then repeat the exercise. Do the entire upper body or lower body workout, THEN repeat the entire workout as a second set, THEN do your cardio or core workout.

WEEK 6: 30 MINUTES PER DAY—CIRCUIT OPTION**
DAY 1: Lower-Body Workout 10 minutes + Second Set of Lower-Body Workout 10 minutes + 30 SECONDS OF CARDIO BETWEEN EACH EXERCISE**
DAY 2: Upper-Body Workout 10 minutes + Core Workout 10 minutes + Second Set of Upper-Body Workout 10 minutes
DAY 3: Lower-Body Workout 10 minutes + Second Set of Lower-Body Workout 10 minutes + 30 SECONDS OF CARDIO BETWEEN EACH EXERCISE**
DAY 4: Upper-Body Workout 10 minutes + Core Workout 10 minutes + Second Set of Upper-Body Workout 10 minutes
DAY 5: Lower-Body Workout 10 minutes + Second Set of Lower-Body Workout 10 minutes + 30 SECONDS OF CARDIO BETWEEN EACH EXERCISE**
DAY 6: Upper-Body Workout 10 minutes + Core Workout 10 minutes + Second Set of Upper-Body Workout 10 minutes
DAY 7: REST

**The option of doing a circuit gives you the opportunity to break up the steady-state cardio days and add some intensity for variety. If you work the 30 seconds of the cardio move intensely, your heart rate will be up higher throughout the entire workout, enhancing your results.

Options abound when you reach this level. You may want to do only the Circuit Option once or twice a week, particularly when you become used to the intensity. You could easily in Week 6 or beyond incorporate the Circuit Option on Monday and on Wednesday do the two sets of Lower-Body Workout, then do steady-state cardio for 10 minutes or longer. Go on a walk or bike ride for a half hour if you have time. On Friday you could go back to your circuit. It's easy to mix and match workouts. If you are short on time and can do only a 10-minute workout, go back to Week 1 and do just one 10-minute workout. It's the consistency that counts. Rather than dropping the entire workout because of time constraints, do a little of something to keep the habit in your body. Results are completely dependent on consistency.

Warm-Up Move: Rhythmic Lunge with Backstroke

Move: Stand with your feet wide. Shift your body weight side to side. When you lunge to the right, backstroke your right arm, with your shoulder blade initiating the move. As you lunge left, backstroke the left arm.

Repetitions: 30 total (15 to the right and 15 to the left).

Tips:

- Feet wide. Do not let your knees jut over your toes in the lunge.
- Feel the ribs open up and the shoulders and shoulder blades move as you make the move bigger.

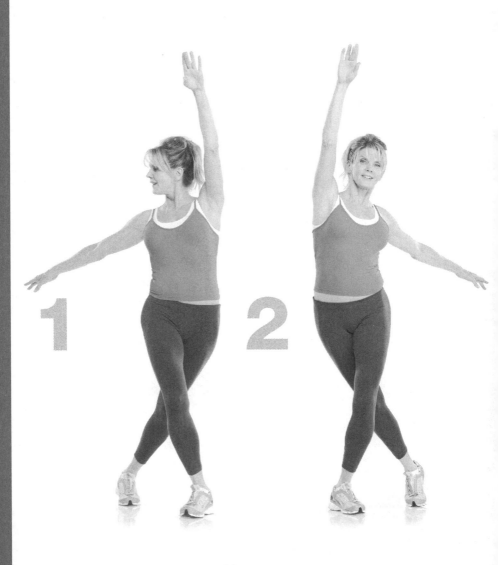

Upper Body

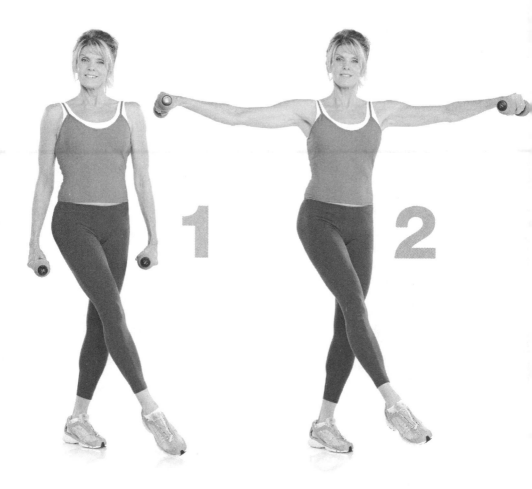

Side Lateral Deltoid Lift with Leg in Rotational Balance

Move: Stand with feet hip distance apart, holding light weights. Lift your right leg and cross it over your left leg. Look toward your right to counter-rotate your torso—lift your spine long as you twist. Lift the weights to shoulder height, squeeze your shoulder blades together, and then lower the weights.

Repetitions: 15 repetitions on each side.

Tips:

- Keep your shoulders down and your shoulder blades together throughout the exercise. Keep your chest open and maintain good posture.
- If the balance aspect is difficult, try tapping your toe on the floor rather than holding it in the air.
- If you feel any discomfort in the shoulders, try turning your palms slightly up.

Upper Body

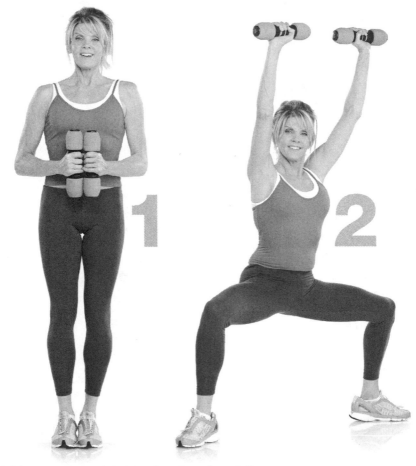

Plié to 4:00 and 8:00 with Overhead Press

Move: Imagine that you are standing in the middle of a clock. Straight in front of you is 12:00 and behind you is 6:00. Step with your right foot, performing a plié, to your right to the 4:00 mark. As you lower into the plié, press weights overhead. Bring the weights back to shoulder level as you return to standing in the middle of your "clock." Alternate stepping to 4:00 and 8:00.

Repetitions: 12 on each side.

Tips:

- Keep your elbows soft as you press the weights overhead.
- Try to drop the hips as low as the knees in your plié. Your hips should not go lower than your knees.
- Step wide enough that the knees are over the ankles in the deepest part of the plié. The knees should not jut over the toes.
- Pull your shoulders back and keep your chest up.
- Pull your abdominal muscles in tight and keep your spine straight.

Hack Squat with Bicep Curls

Move: Stand with feet hip distance apart. Hold medium to heavy weights.
Lift your left foot and then drive the heel out, placing it on the floor about
12 inches in front of your right foot. Sit back into the hack squat by pushing
your hips behind you, keeping your chest up. As you come out of the squat,
do a bicep curl.

Repetitions: 12 on each side.

Tips:

• Keep your chest up, shoulders back, and abdominal muscles in.
• Really sit back into the back heel—do not let weight drift into your toes.
• As you sit into the squat, be aware of feeling the stretch in the front leg.

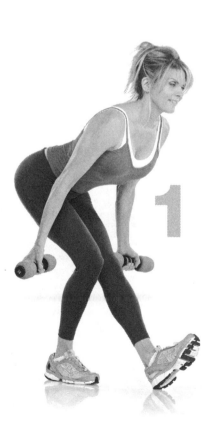
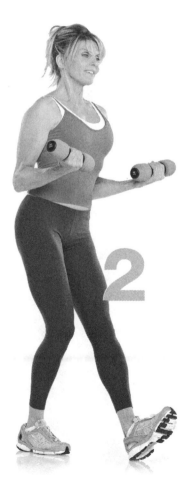

Tricep Kickback and Posterior Deltoid Lift in a Squat

Move: Hold light to medium weights. Stand with your feet hip width apart and bend your knees, driving your hips back into a squat. Tuck your elbows into your waist, then straighten your elbows behind you. Then lift the straight arms. As you bend your elbows back in, return to standing.

Repetitions: 15 total.

Tips:
- In the squat sit back into your heels.
- Control the weights. Do not allow them to have momentum or swing.
- Aim your elbows high in the tricep press.
- Keep your shoulders back, chest up and open, and spine straight.
- Pull your navel toward your spine.

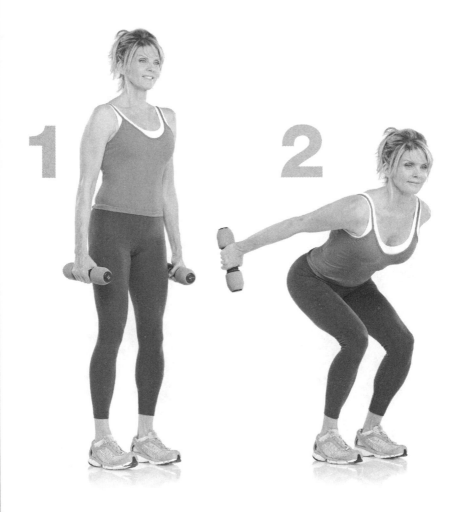

Upper Body

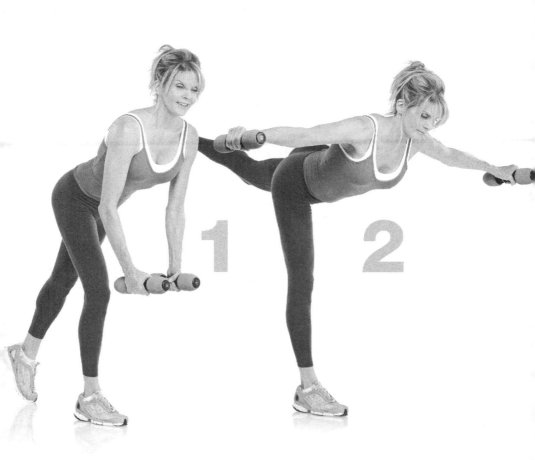

Back Flye with Balance

Move: Stand on your right leg, holding light weights. Lift your left leg off the floor behind you and balance. Start with your hands directly under your body, palms facing each other, then lift the weights and squeeze the shoulder blades together.

Repetitions: 12 on each side.

Tips:

- Keep your chest lifted as you balance.
- Your may feel this more in your standing leg than your lifted leg.
- If balancing is difficult for you, tap your foot on the floor.
- Lift the weights with control. Squeeze your shoulder blades together as you finish the move.
- Keep your abdominal muscles pulled up and in.

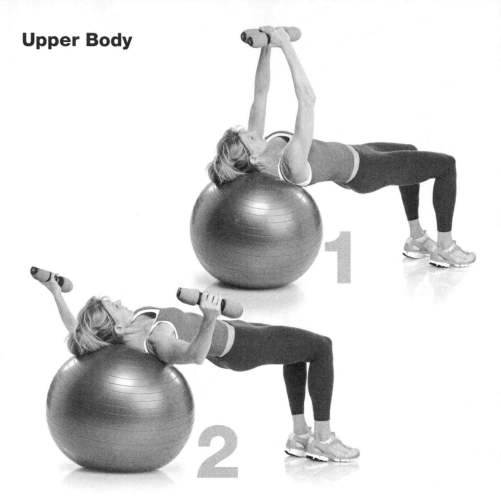

Chest Flye and Press on the Ball

Move: Sit on a ball, holding medium weights. Roll out until your shoulder blades touch the ball. Squeeze your glutes to lift your hips and rest your head on the ball. Hold the weights over your chest, hands turned so your palms are facing. As the weights go down into a flye, squeeze your shoulder blades together. To do a chest press, turn the weights so they are end to end. Bring the weights down, engaging the shoulder blades, and then press them back up.

Repetitions: 12 chest flyes and 12 chest presses.

Tips:
- Knit your ribs together and pull the navel in toward the spine. Do not let your back arch.
- Use your glutes to press your hips up. Don't let the hips drop.
- Stay in control when doing flyes and presses. Do not let your weights sink lower than your shoulders. Keep the muscles active.
- Squeeze the shoulder blades together to anchor the upper back when the weights are in the lowest position.
- If you do not have a stability ball, use a dense pillow so your torso is slightly above the floor.

Tricep Extension on the Ball

Move: Roll out on the ball as you did for chest flyes and presses. Bring the weights over your head, bending your elbows until the weights just barely tap the ball. Keep your upper arms at that angle as you straighten and bend your elbows.

Repetitions: 12 to 15.

Tips:

- Do not let your back arch. Tuck your pelvis slightly and keep the abdominal muscles active.
- Keep your elbows over your forehead. Do not let them move as you do the presses.
- If your shoulder muscles are tight, you may not be able to tap the ball. Lower the weights as close to the ball as you can, staying within a range of motion that is comfortable for your body.

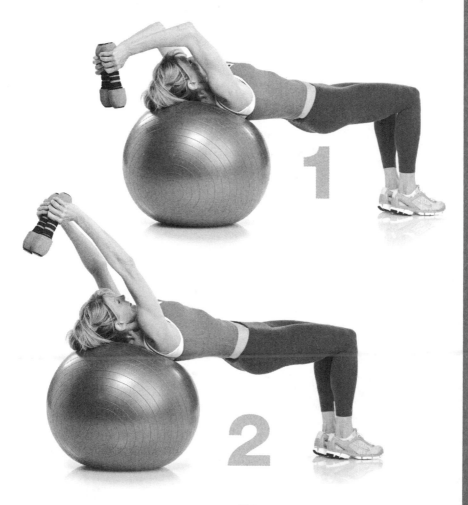

Push-Up

Move: Lying facedown on the floor, place your hands under your shoulders, tucking your toes underneath you. Push up into a plank. Keep your abdominal muscles lifted up toward your spine. If this is too difficult, drop your knees to the floor, modifying the push-up. Have your hands pointed slightly inward. Lower yourself toward the floor, trying to achieve about a 90 degree bend in the elbows. Exhale as you press back up. Repeat with the left leg lifted.

Repetitions: 12 on each side.

Tips:

- Keep your abdominal muscles contracted. Knitting your rib cage together will help to keep the lower back from sagging.
- If your core is weak, you may need to move to a modified push-up because the push-up from your toes is more difficult not only for your chest, arms and back but also for your core. If your back is not straight, your rib cage cannot stay knit together. If you feel any discomfort in your lower back, modify the push-up by dropping down to your knees.

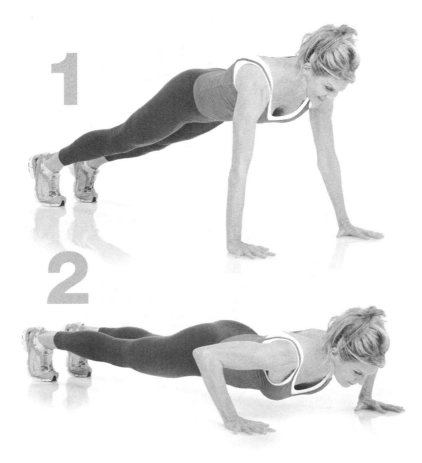

Upper Body

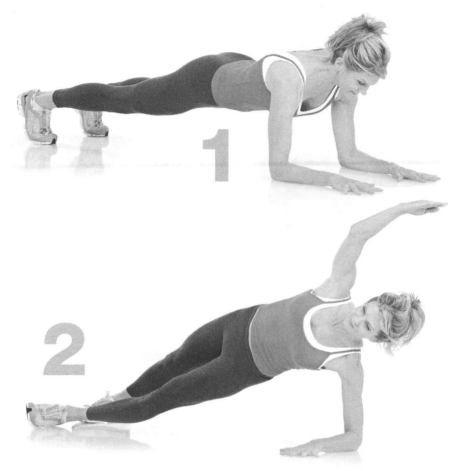

Rolling Plank T-Stand on Forearms

Move: Start in a modified push-up position with your forearms and feet on the floor. Have your feet about 12 inches apart. Pull the navel in toward the spine and keep it there as you breathe in and out for about 15 seconds. Roll to your right forearm, turning both your feet onto their sides. With your left arm in the air, squeeze the shoulder blades together, opening your chest. Hold this for 15 seconds. Then roll to the left forearm, lifting your right arm into the air. Squeeze the shoulder blades together again and open the chest. Hold for 15 seconds.

Repetitions: 1 in the plank, 1 on right forearm, 1 on left forearm.

Tips:

- Keep your abdominal muscles lifted and your navel pulled in toward your spine.
- Hips should stay lifted when rolling to a side.
- Pull the shoulder blades together when you lift one arm off the floor.
- As you do these moves, keep your body stiff and tight in the position.

Lower Body

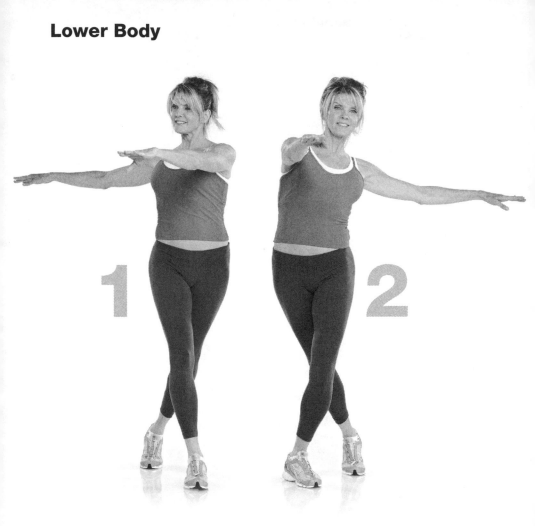

Warm-Up—Step Touch with Cross-Back Leg and Opposition Arms

Move: To warm up your body, step side to side, tapping your leg diagonally behind you while reaching the same arm as leg to the front. Gradually make the movement bigger.

Repetitions: 30 on each side.

Tips:

- Stand erect, shoulders back, chest up, and head lifted tall. Pull your abdominal muscles in.
- Stretch your arm forward and your leg back in opposition, feeling the mild stretch through the torso.
- Adding propulsion can increase the intensity of the move. Propulsion can be added by simply leaping out of the tap, landing softly into the next step.

Squat with Side Lift and Overhead Press

Move: Stand with your feet hip width apart and hold weights at shoulder level. Sit back and lower your hips, bending your knees to about a 90-degree angle. As you return to a standing position, lift your right leg, pressing the left arm overhead. Repeat on the other side.

Repetitions: 12 on each side.

Tips:

- Drive your hips back, keeping your weight in your heels. Your weight should never shift onto your toes.
- Keep your chest up. Do not arch or round the back.
- As your leg lifts, squeeze the muscles around the hip. Rather than focus on lifting your leg high, increase the intensity by aiming the leg low.
- As you press the weight overhead, maintain a slight bend in the elbow.

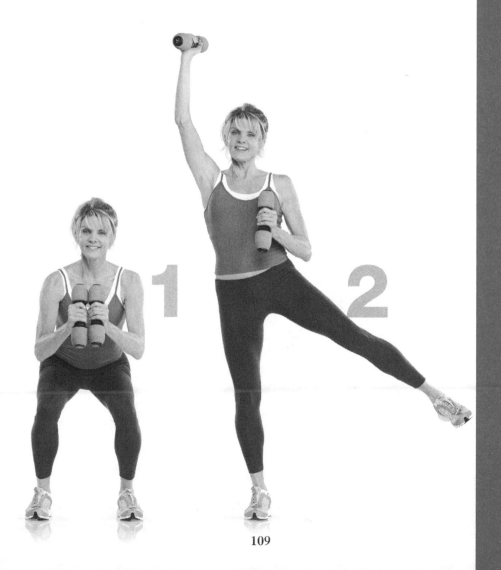

Step-Back Lunge with Cross Chop

Move: Reach your arms diagonally across your body to the left as you step back with your right leg and dip into a lunge. Pull your arms across your body to the right hip as you slide your right leg back to standing.

Repetitions: 12 on each side.

Tips:

- Step back far enough into the lunge so that the front knee is directly over the front ankle.
- When your arms reach diagonally above your shoulder, hold your core muscles tight to keep the lower back from arching.
- The move can be done with a towel or weights.
- For a challenge lift your knee toward your chest, balancing on one foot instead of coming just to standing.

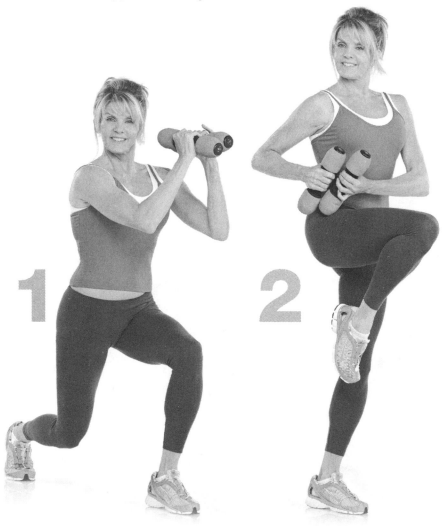

Lower Body

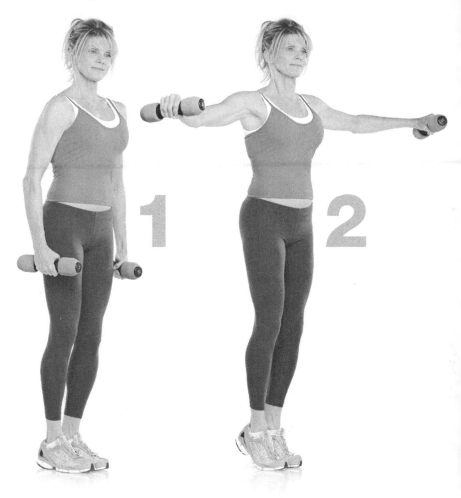

Calf Raises with Side Lateral Lift

Move: Stand tall with feet together, holding medium to light weights by your sides. Lift up onto your toes, lifting the weights laterally to shoulder height. Pull your shoulder blades together and then lower the weights slowly as you lower yourself from your toes to a standing position.

Repetitions: 12 to 15.

Tips:

- Keep your shoulders back and chest up. Always work on your posture before performing the move.
- Pull your shoulder blades together at the top of the move and control the weights as you lower them.
- Calf raises can be performed on a stair for more intensity.
- If the lateral raise bothers your shoulders, try turning your palms slightly upward.

Lower Body

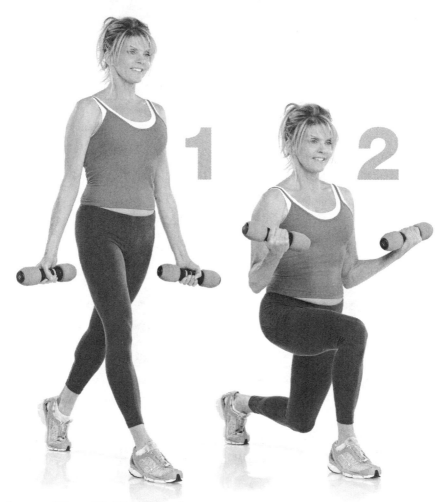

Lunge Dip with Bicep Curl

Move: Stand with your feet parallel, hip distance apart, holding a medium to heavy weight in each hand. Step back with your left leg and dip into a lunge. As you dip down bend your elbows, performing a bicep curl. Keeping your back straight, dip straight down and up.

Repetitions: 12 with the right leg in front and 12 with the left leg in front.

Tips:

- Step back far enough into the lunge so that the front knee stays over the ankle as you dip down. The front knee should not drift forward over your toes.
- Keep your shoulders over your hips—do not lean forward.
- Your hip can go down as low as your knee (about a 90-degree bend of the knee).
- As you bicep curl keep your elbows directly underneath your shoulders.

Penny in the Pocket with a One-Arm Row

Move: Stand tall with your body weight on your right foot. Place your left foot on the floor behind the right, keeping your weight on the right foot. Pretend there is a penny on the floor. Bend over to pick it up using your right arm, then stand up and put it in your "pocket."

Repetitions: 15 with the right leg forward and 15 with the left leg forward.

Tips:

- Beginners should try this move without a weight. Slowly incorporate a light weight.
- Keep your spine straight. Do not curve your back.
- Keep your weight on your front foot. Try to either very lightly tap the floor with your back foot or hover it off the floor.

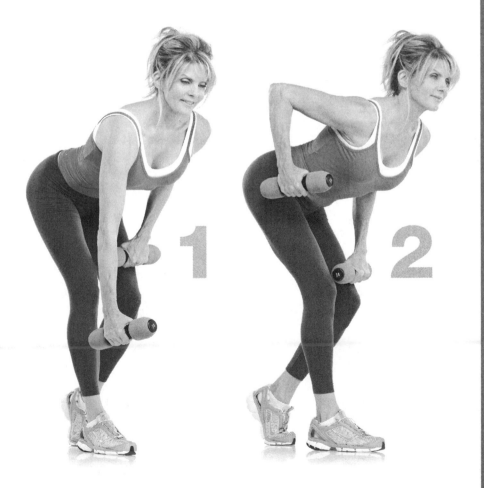

One-Legged Squatting Dead Lift with Back Row

Move: Put your right foot about 12 inches in front of your left. Keep your spine straight and hinge over at the hips. Lower your hips toward the floor, keeping your body weight on the right heel. As you lower your hips, pull weights up with your elbows just brushing your waist. Return to starting position and repeat.

Repetitions: 12 with the right leg forward and 12 with the left leg forward. As you become stronger try to do this exercise with no weight on the back foot. When you perform the back row, finish the move by squeezing the shoulder blades together.

Tips:

- Keep your body weight in the front heel. Do not let it drift into the front toes.
- Keep your back straight and your chest lifted. Do not round your spine.
- As you get stronger do this exercise with no weight on the back foot.

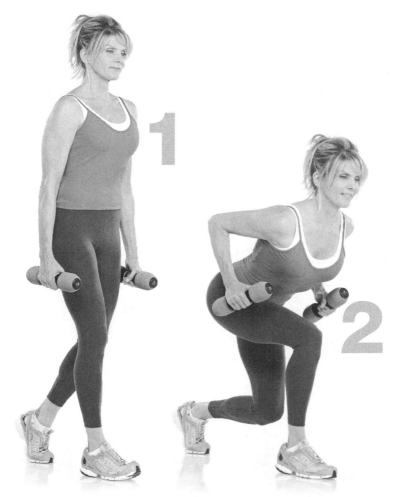

Lower Body

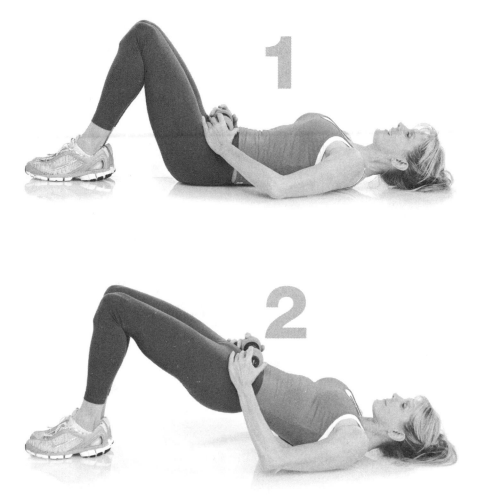

Bridge with Weights on Hips

Move: Lie on your back with knees bent. Hold a light to medium weight on the crease between the leg and the hips. Lift your hips off the floor. Lift your right leg off the floor and then lift and lower the hips 15 times. Repeat with your left leg off the floor.

Repetitions: 15 on each side.

Tips:
- In the bridge keep your thighs, hips, and ribs in a straight line.
- Keep your abdominal muscles pulled in.
- If the exercise is too difficult, do it with both feet on the floor.

Lower Body

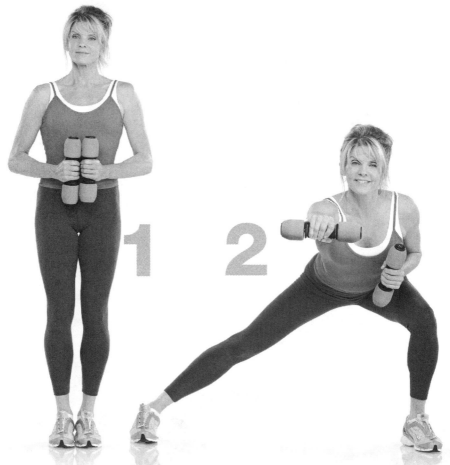

Lunge to 9:00 and 3:00, Reaching Forward

Move: Stand with feet together, holding a light weight in each hand. Take a wide step to the right, pressing the weight in your left hand in front of your body at shoulder height. Return to starting position, then lunge to the left, pressing the weight in your right hand in front of your body at shoulder height.

Repetitions: 12 on each side.

Tips:

- Make sure your stance is wide enough. Your knee should be over the ankle in the lowest part of the lunge.
- As you drop your hips into the lunge, keep your weight in your heel. Do not let your weight shift into your toes.
- Keep your chest open and your shoulders back.

Squat with Rotating Twist

Move: Stand with feet hip distance apart, holding light weights in each hand. Push your hips back until your knees are bent to about a 90-degree angle, pulling weights to the chest. As you rise keep the left foot and hip parallel but pivot on the right toe, turning your whole body to the left. As you pivot on the right toe, squeeze the right glute while bringing the weights overhead toward your left side.

Repetitions: 12 with your right toe pivoting and 12 with your left.

Tips:

- As you squat sit back into your heels and keep your chest up.
- As you pivot squeeze your glute.
- As the weights go overhead make sure that you remain in control. Do not let your back arch or round. Keep your core braced.

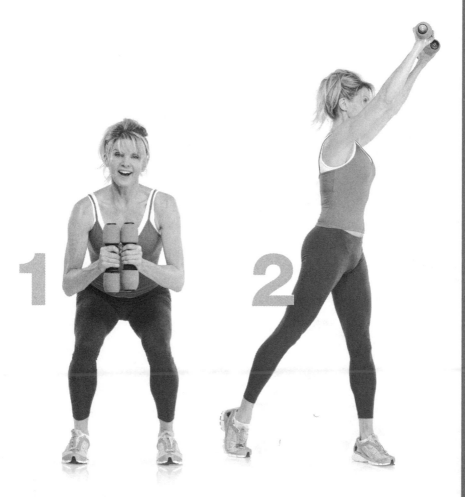

Crunch on the Ball

Move: Sit on the ball, then roll out by walking your feet away from the ball until they are under your knees. Place your hands behind your head, supporting your head and neck. Lift your shoulders off the ball by sliding your ribs down toward the top of your pelvis. As you go back down, do not release the ribs, but slide them back toward their original position with control. During all phases of the movement, pull your navel toward your spine.

Repetitions: 20 total.

Tips:

- Slide the rib cage down toward the top of the pelvis and squeeze the abdominal muscles to finish the move.
- Placing your hips higher up on the ball is harder. Lower is easier.
- Feet closer together is harder. Feet wider apart is easier.
- If you do not have a ball, do these crunches on the floor.

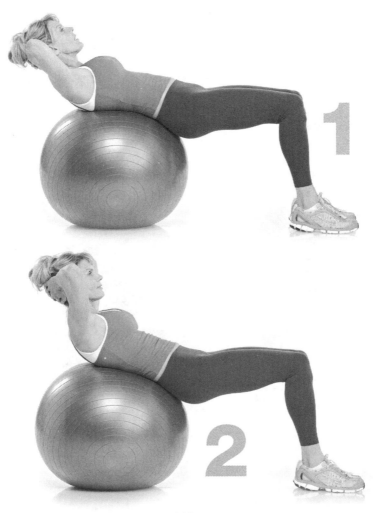

Core

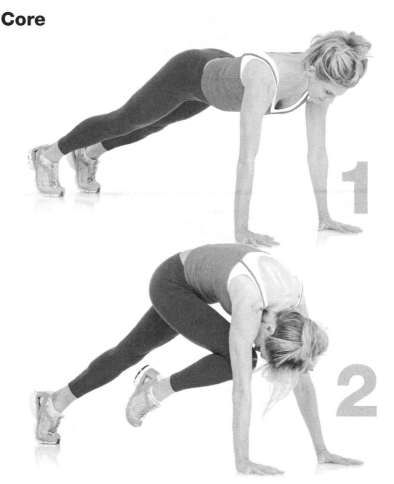

Tuck in Plank, Optional Swivel Under

Move: Go into a plank position with hands and feet on the floor. Pull the right knee in toward your chest, keeping your hips low. Lean into your arms as you tuck, bringing the knee all the way to your elbow. Repeat with the left knee, alternating right and left.

Repetitions: 12 tucks on each side.

Optional Swivel Under: Pull your right knee into your chest; swivel the left foot, bringing your right knee under you to your left. Lift your right tucked knee as high as you can. Finish by tucking the knee to your chest and then place it back on the floor, bracing your core muscles. Repeat with the left knee tucked and swiveled under.

Repetitions: 8 swivels each side.

Tips:
- Your body should start in a straight line. Do not let your hips sag or pop up.
- Do not swing the knee toward your chest; squeeze it in.
- When you swivel squeeze the knee up in a tuck. Do not swing it up.
- Beginners can work up to this exercise by first mastering the moves on forearms and knees.

Core

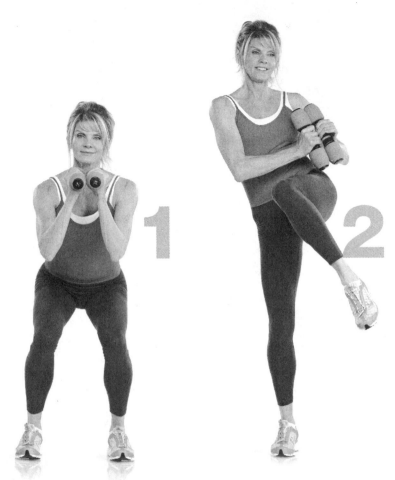

Squat with Cross Chop

Move: Stand with feet hip width apart. Hold a light to medium weight in each hand. Push your hips back into a squat, sitting back into your heels. As you return to standing, bring your right knee up toward your chest on the left side and bring the weights toward the right hip. Repeat the squat, lifting your left knee, chopping with the weights to the left hip.

Repetitions: 12 on each side.

Tips:

- When doing the squat keep your chest up, sit back into your heels, and drop to a 90-degree bend of the knee.
- When doing the chop keep your spine straight. Do not round your back.
- Use a squeeze rather than momentum to do the move.

Discus Thrower

Move: Stand with feet hip width apart, holding a light weight in each hand. Push your hips back into a squat and hold the weight in your right hand near your right ankle. As you rise keep the left foot parallel (do not let it pivot or move sideways), but pivot on the right toe, squeezing the right glute, turning your hips to face the left. As you do this, sweep the weight in a fluid motion from your feet, up and out, until it is over your head on the left.

Repetitions: 12 on each side.

Tips:

- Chest up—do not collapse your spine as you squat.
- Sit back into your heels in the squat, attempting to bend your knees to a 90-degree angle.
- This move also works well with a ball or weighted medicine ball.
- As the weights sweep overhead, make sure that you remain under control. Do not let your back arch or round and keep your core muscles braced.

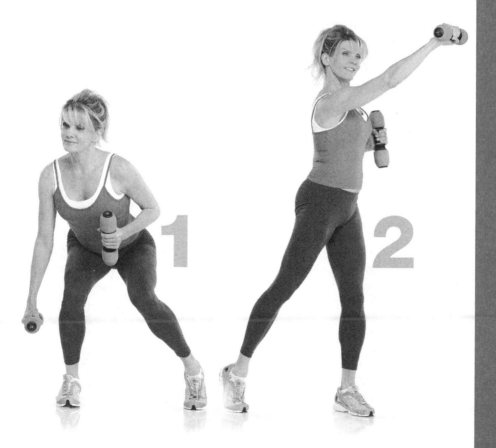

Bump

Move: Stand tall with feet together. Begin by letting your hips rock to the right, keeping your feet together. As you get your rhythm going, step out with the right foot, still bumping your hips out to the right. Progress into the move by adding the right arm overhead as you step away with the leg.

Repetitions: 12 on each side.

Tips:

- Keep your abdominal muscles pulled in. Do not let your back arch or slump.
- Start the move with no weights in your hands. Work up to using light weights.

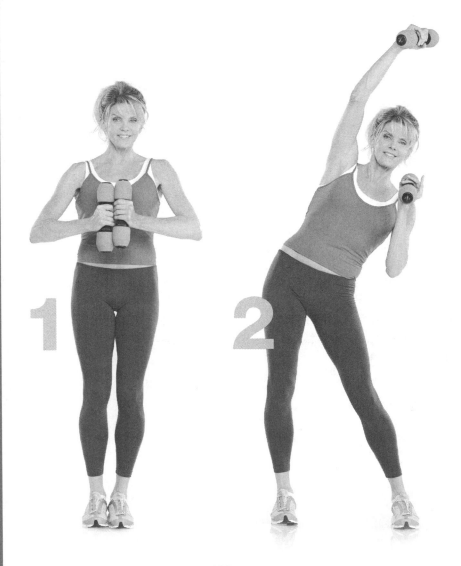

Core

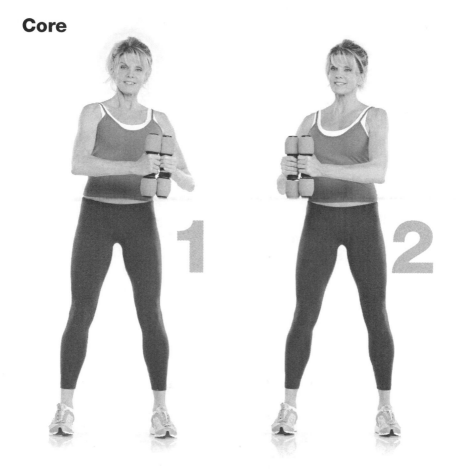

Standing Twist/Rotation to 10:00 and 2:00

Move: Stand tall with feet 2 to 3 feet apart. Slightly bend your knees. Place your hands together in front of your stomach. Squeeze your glutes and inner thigh muscles to anchor and brace your lower body. Pull your shoulder blades together and tightly pull in your abdominal muscles. Twist your upper body side to side. If you were standing on the middle of a clock, your torso would rotate to face the 10:00 mark and the 2:00 mark.

Repetitions: 15 on each side.

Tips:

- Pay close attention to your posture. Keep your shoulders back, your chest lifted, your abdominal muscles pulled in, and your spine long.
- For more intensity in the legs, you can drop your hips until they are almost as low as your knees. In this position be sure your knees are over your ankles, not forward over your toes.
- Twist only as far as you can without moving your lower body. 10:00 and 2:00 are guidelines.
- All the movement is from the waist up. Keep your hips still.
- This exercise is done without weights. Light weights can be added if you keep the exercise slow and under control.

Core

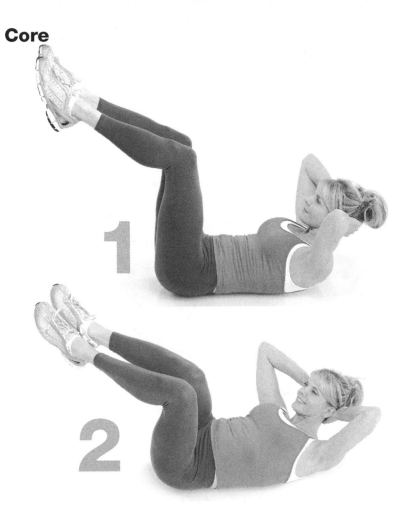

Crunching Tabletop—Straight and Swivel

Move: Lie on your back, knees over hips (tabletop position). Lift your shoulders into a crunch, squeezing the abdominal muscles. Bring your shoulders down, keeping tension on the muscle.

Repetitions: 20 total.

To swivel, place your hands behind your head and reach your right elbow toward your right ankle as you crunch, swiveling your knees toward the left. Repeat on the other side.

Repetitions: 12 on each side.

Tips:

- When you swivel keep your feet and knees together and swivel them as one unit. Feel your ribs slide down toward the hips on the side you are working. The more you swivel the feet, the more you should feel the oblique muscles. Try not to move your knees into a tuck, but stay in a tabletop position.
- The move becomes more intense when your knees are farther away from your chest. If your spine arches off the floor (a form break), pull your knees back in toward your chest to decrease intensity.

Kayaking

Move: Sit upright with your knees bent, feet on the floor, chest lifted. Lift your feet off the floor, balancing on your sacrum, tucking your knees into your chest. Place your hands on the floor by your hips. Swivel your knees side to side. Advanced option: Lift your hands off the floor and move the arms in opposition to the legs. As the knees and legs drop to the right, your hands and elbows will aim at your left hip.

Repetitions: 30 total.

Tips:

- Keep your chest lifted and your spine straight. Do not slump.
- Start the progression with your hands on the floor. As you get stronger try moving side to side with your hands moving hip to hip. Beginners may want to start with the balance and no swivel.

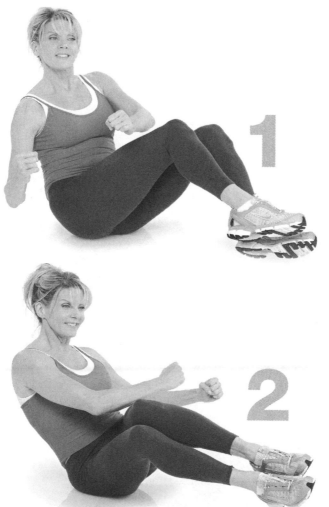

Double Leg Stretch

Move: Lie on your back with your knees tucked into your chest, head and shoulders up off the floor, and hands reaching beyond toward feet. As you inhale push your legs out away from your center and reach one arm overhead, keeping the other arm bent behind your head and your shoulders and head up. Exhale as you return to your tuck position.

Repetitions: 12 total.

Tips:

- Your head, shoulders, and shoulder blades are up off the floor in both phases of the exercise—in the tuck and when you open out.
- Your lower back should not arch off the floor when you open out of the tuck. If it does you have broken form and need to decrease the intensity. Make the movement smaller and open up less.
- Beginners will tuck, and when they open up, their feet should be over the hips and the hands should be right over the shoulders.
- Keep your shoulders down and away from your ears. Press the shoulder blades down deep in the back to keep the neck long.
- Pull the navel toward the spine throughout the exercise.

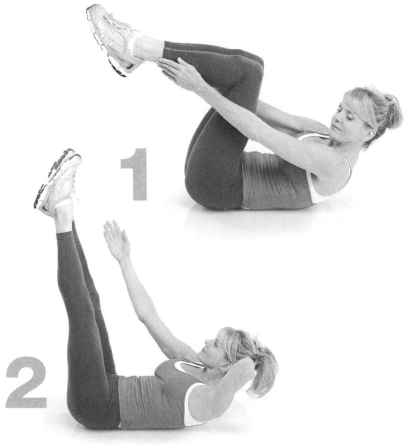

Core

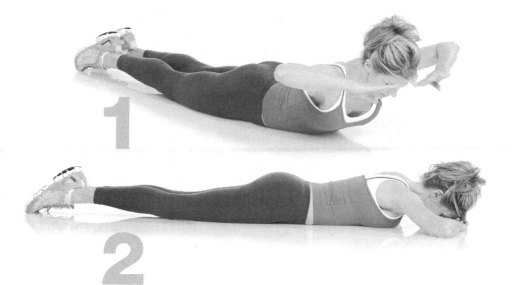

Hyperextension/House for a Mouse

Move: Lie face down on the floor. Keeping the ribs and pubic bone on the floor, pull your navel up off the floor.

Another way to do this exercise is to move into it from a hyperextension. Start lying prone with your hands on the floor by your shoulders. Lift your body up just enough so you have your legs and pubic bone on the floor, but the rest of the torso is hovering off the floor. Pull your navel toward the spine and start to lower your body. Imagine having the next thing that touches the floor be your ribs, not your navel area—while keeping your pubic bone on the floor. This activation of the abdominal muscles creates a "House for a Mouse."

Place your hands near your shoulders. Keep your "House for a Mouse" and lift your upper body off the floor. Next try lifting only your legs off the floor, continuing to hold your "House for a Mouse." Finish with both upper and lower body lifting together, always trying to keep the "House for a Mouse."

Repetitions: 8 with upper body lifting, 8 with lower body lifting, and 8 with both upper and lower body lifting off the floor.

Tips:

- Your pubic bone and lower ribs are your anchors. Your body will rest on these bones while the muscle between these bones (the transverse abdominis) activates, pulling the navel toward the spine (away from the floor).
- If you pull the abs away from the floor properly, your body will not lift up very high when you do the upper body and lower body repetitions.
- If your abs do not actually lift high enough to come off the floor and make space for a mouse, that's OK. The focus is to activate the abdominals and move the belly button up and in, no matter how small the movement—even if the movement does not actually lift the belly off the floor.

Cardio

The following cardio moves will add intensity to your Matrix routines and get your heart rate up higher for a longer burn. Starting in Week 3 (or Week 2 in the advanced version), you'll inject these cardio "blasts" in between your Matrix moves, adding about 10 extra minutes to the workout. For live video of these moves in action, go to my website.

Jogging in Place
Move: As you jog the ball of the foot will land on the floor first and then your heel should drop to the floor.
Tips:
- Be fluid. Land softly on your feet.
- For more intensity try adding Mountain Climber Arms. As your foot strikes the floor, the same arm drives up high.

Cross-Country Skiing
Move: Rebound landing on both feet simultaneously, with one foot forward and the other back.
Tips:
- As you land sink into your legs, feeling the shock absorption of the knees and hips.
- This move can be done slowly with the emphasis on shock absorption or quickly as you rebound from right lead to left lead.

Alternating Knee Repeater with Knee Chop
Move: Stand on your left leg and bring your right knee toward your chest on the left side of your body. As you do your arms will chop to the knee, meeting it. Repeat this move for 30 to 60 seconds. Then repeat the move standing on your right leg, pulling in the left knee.
Tips:
- Add a little twist by letting your arms go to the outside of the right knee.
- For more intensity in the move, when standing on your right leg, put your weight into your right heel so that you can drop your hips lower.
- Rapidly pull the knee in and out, chopping with the arms for up to one minute.

Side-to-Side Tap Behind with Leap
Move: Step to the right, then tap the floor behind your right foot with your left foot. Then step to the left and tap the floor with your right foot. Increase the intensity by leaping from side to side. Repeat this move for one minute.
Tip:
- Try to cross your inner thighs as you bring your foot behind; don't just cross your foot behind.

Hip Hike
Move:
Balance on your right leg and lift your left knee toward your left armpit.
As your knee goes up, your left elbow and arm will chop down to meet it.
Switch to the other leg. Repeat the move for 30 seconds, then switch to the
other side.
Tip:
• As you repeat the move, hike the hip of the moving leg toward the rib cage.

Boxer Shuffle on the Clock
Move: Imagine you are standing on a clock at 12:00. A boxer shuffle is a
bouncy move shifting your weight from right foot to left foot. Leading with
the right leg, take the right foot to 1:00, 2:00, 3:00, 4:00, 5:00, and 6:00,
moving back up and down the clock, keeping your left foot at 12:00.
Repeat moving your left foot down the clock to 11:00, 10:00, 9:00, 8:00,
7:00, and 6:00. Shuffle each side of the clock for 30 seconds.
Tip:
• To learn the boxer shuffle, try jogging in place slowly, keeping your feet
  closer and closer to the floor. Widen your feet as you do this small jog
  and you should end up in a boxer shuffle.

Power Down/Step Touch and Stick
Move: Starting on both feet, laterally leap to the right, landing on your right
foot and absorbing your body weight with your hips and knees. Step back
to your left and repeat the leap to the right. As you do the move, twist your
torso to the right, reaching out with your arms, sticking the move. Leap
30 seconds to the right and then repeat leaping 30 seconds to the left.
Tip:
• Land softly from the leap as you stick the move.

Step Touch Ham Curl
Move: Step to the right, lifting your left foot up toward your left glute, then
step to the left, lifting the right foot toward the right glute. As you lift your
foot, pull your elbows toward your waist and squeeze your shoulder blades
together. Repeat side to side for one minute.
Tip.
• Advanced exercisers can add propulsion by leaping from side to side
  with a soft landing, or they can make the move bouncy.

Jump Rope

Move: This move can be done with or without a jump rope. If you do not have one, mimic the jump rope move with either a small hop, a small jog, or by skipping. Other variations include using your feet in a cross-country fashion: one in front of the other as you jump from foot to foot. Or try double jumps: jumping two narrow, two wide, or one foot at a time.

Tip:
- Land softly. Keep your feet fluid. Land on the ball of your foot and absorb your weight as you lower onto your heel.

Happy Feet

Move: Start with a small jog and then double-time the feet so that they are going as fast as they can go as close to the floor as possible.

Tip:
- Do the move for a whole minute or in intervals of 15 to 30 seconds with some recovery between intervals.

Twisties

Move: Hop and land on both feet, swiveling right and left as you hop. Use your arms to counter-rotate through the waist.

Tips:
- Land softly.
- Stay in control through the arms as you twist.

Stretching

The following 12 stretches give you a full body routine. You can use them in a variety of ways, choosing to do all of them or just a few that target areas you have worked the most on a given day. You will likely find favorites that you use every day. Try to stretch your whole body by going through all 12 stretches at least twice a week.

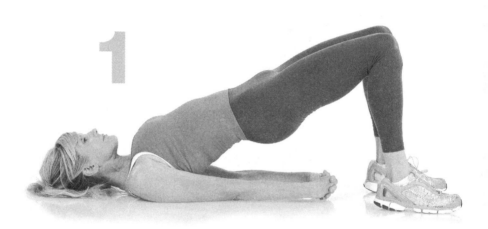

Bridge

Move: Lie on your back with your knees bent and your feet under your knees. Have your hands by your sides next to your hips. Inhale, expanding your ribs. As you exhale begin knitting the ribs together, pressing your lower back into the floor. As you do tilt the tailbone off the floor and start to lift your vertebrae off the floor one by one from the tailbone upward until you are up to your shoulder blades. Bring your arms underneath you, lacing your fingers together. Rock from side to side a little to reach your hands down farther toward your feet, opening the neck and shoulders. Hold the stretch for about 20 to 30 seconds.

Tips:
- Keep the ribs knit together. Do not let the ribs open, which will create an arch in the lower back.
- Press your feet into the floor, keeping your hips lifted.
- When you draw your hands under you, with your fingers laced together open the chest and lengthen your neck.

Stretching

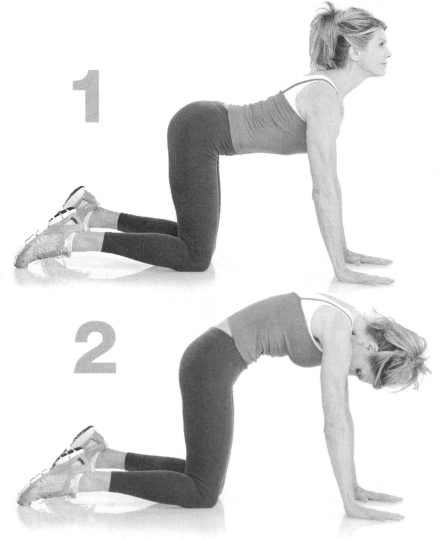

Cat/Dog

Move: Kneel on your hands and knees, hips over knees and shoulders over wrists. Pull your navel toward your spine, rounding your back and feeling the stretch in the lower back. Hold this stretch for 20 seconds. Then lift your chest and your tailbone, feeling the back arch. Hold for 20 seconds.

Tips:

- Stay within the range of motion that feels comfortable for your body. Do not overstretch.
- If either of these stretches bothers your lower back, try shortening the range of motion.
- For variety try shrugging the right shoulder slightly to feel more stretch on the right side of your spine, then repeat on the left.

Spinal Twist

Move: Lie on your back with your knees bent, feet underneath knees. Stretch your arms to the sides with palms at shoulder height. Drop your knees toward your right side, crossing your knees one on top of the other. Keep both shoulder blades down. Your head and neck will be in alignment with your shoulders facing up. To exit the move, draw your top knee up to your chest and let your other leg follow. Give yourself a full breath or two before beginning the stretch on the other side. Hold the stretch for 20 to 30 seconds on each side.

Tips:

- Always stay within a comfortable range of motion. You should feel a gentle tug. Avoid overstretching.
- Keep your shoulders, neck, and upper body muscles relaxed.
- Use your breath. As you exhale sink deeper into the stretch.

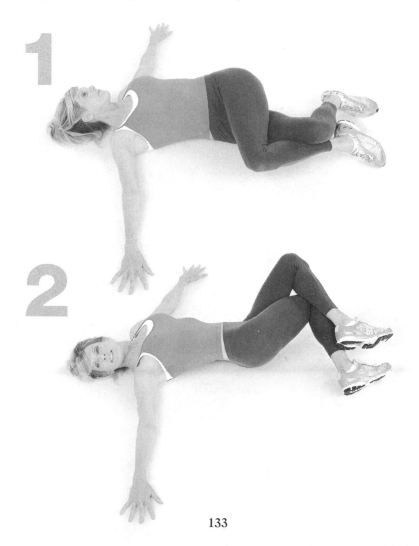

Hamstring Straddle

Move: Sit on the floor with your feet in front of you. Move your feet into the widest "V" that you can comfortably make. Sit tall. Do not slump your spine forward. Keep your spine straight and your chest lifted. Lean forward until you feel a tug in the back of the thighs. Hold the stretch for 20 to 30 seconds.

Tips:

- If you flex your feet in this position, you will also feel a calf stretch.
- Stretch to the point of a mild pull. Do not overstretch.
- If you cannot sit up straight before starting the stretch, put your hands behind your hips to help you sit more upright rather than having your hands on the floor in front of you. You could also sit on a pillow or bolster to raise your hips. This will make the stretch easier.

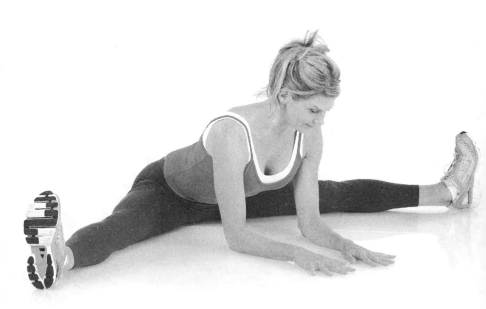

Stretching

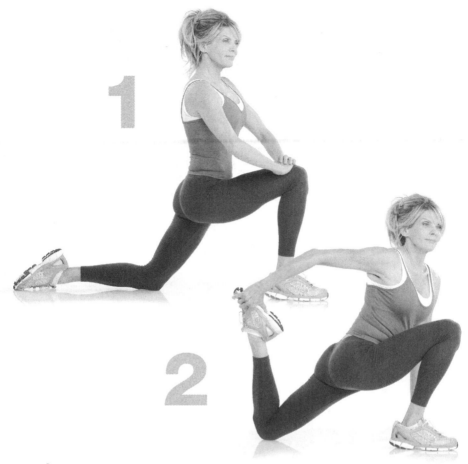

Lunge

Move 1: With your left foot in front and your right leg back in the lunge, drop your right knee to the floor on a padded surface such as a pillow, folded towel, or yoga mat. Reach around to your right and grab your right foot, bringing it closer to your right glute. Do not let your right hip pop up when you bring the foot in closer. Hold for 20 to 30 seconds, then repeat on other side.

Move 2: From a standing position bend over and put your hands on the floor, one hand on either side of your left foot. Take a very large step back with your right leg. Keep your right knee straight, drop your hips, and make sure that your left knee is over your left ankle. Reach the right heel back and squeeze the right glute to intensify the stretch in the hip flexor. Repeat with the left leg behind you. Hold each side for 20 to 30 seconds.

Tips:

- Make sure you step back far enough into the lunge. When you are in the stretch, the front knee should be over the front ankle.
- Keep your chest up, shoulders back, and posture intact during both stretches.

Butterfly

Move: Sit on the floor. Keep your spine straight and draw your heels together. Let your knees drop to the sides. Place your hands on your feet with the thumbs on the insides of your feet. Open up the soles of the feet as if you were opening a book. Your elbows can press your knees open at this point if you like. Use your breath to open the stretch. Hold the stretch for 20 to 30 seconds.

Tips:

• Sit up tall. Keep your chest up and your spine straight.
• If you cannot lean forward into the stretch, it is fine to keep your hands behind your hips and use them to press your body forward.
• If you find it hard to sit up straight, try sitting on a firm pillow to raise your hips a couple of inches off the floor.

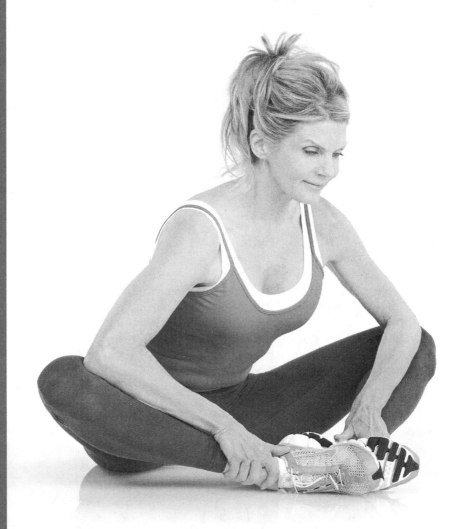

Stretching

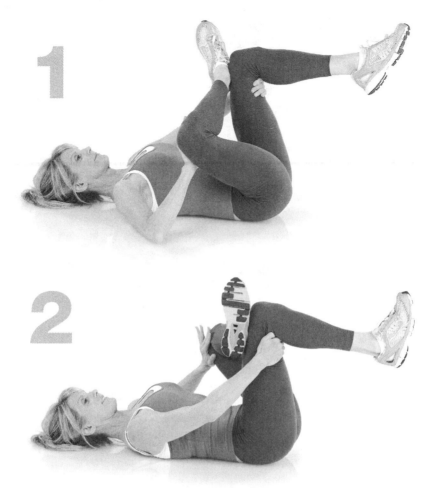

Figure Four

Move: Lie on your back with your feet on the floor and your knees bent. Draw your right knee up to your chest, then rotate it out to the right so that your right foot is directly over your chest. Pull your left leg up off the floor and put your right foot on the left thigh, right above the left knee. Use your left hand to help pull the left thigh inward and use your right hand to push the right knee away from you. You should feel a stretch in your right hip. Hold the stretch for 20 to 30 seconds. Repeat with your left leg.

Tips:

- Remain even on both hips while doing the stretch. Do not lean on one hip more than the other.
- If you slide the foot that is on your thigh closer to the hip or move it closer to the knee, it will change the angle of the stretch. If you experiment with this, make sure you do it on both sides.

Stretching

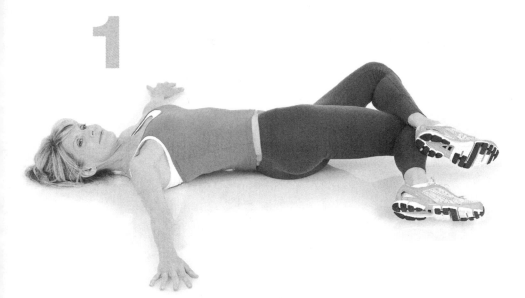

Piriformis Stretch in an "X"

Move: Lie on your back with your legs flat. Bring the left knee inward, crossing it under the right knee and making an "X" with your legs. Drop the left leg toward the floor. You should feel most of the intensity in the right hip. Repeat with the left leg on top. Hold each stretch for 20 to 30 seconds.

Tip:
- If you find that one side is tighter than the other, either stretch the tighter side with more intensity or stretch it a second time to work to create similar flexibility on each side.

Triceps Stretch

Move: Sit, kneel, or stand tall. Lift your right arm overhead. Bend your elbow, aiming it toward the ceiling. Use your left hand to pull the right elbow back, stretching the tricep muscles. Hold the stretch on each side for 20 to 30 seconds.

Tips:

- Keep your head tall when performing the stretch. Do not let it bow forward.
- Keep your abdominal muscles pulled inward.

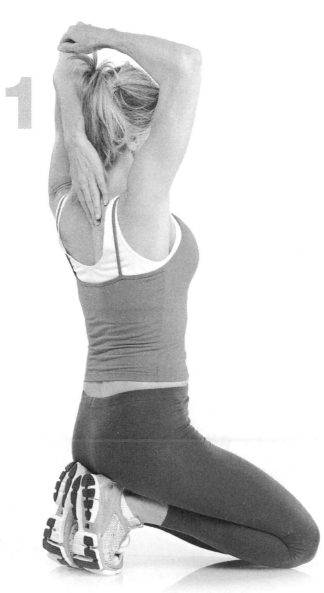

Chest Opener Seated

Move: Sit or stand tall. Clasp your hands behind your back. Holding your hands or fingers, open your chest by pulling the shoulder blades together, lifting the arms up behind you. Hold the stretch for 20 to 30 seconds.

Tips:

- Keep your shoulders pressed down. Do not let the shoulders shrug upward during the stretch.
- Squeeze your shoulder blades toward your spine during the stretch.

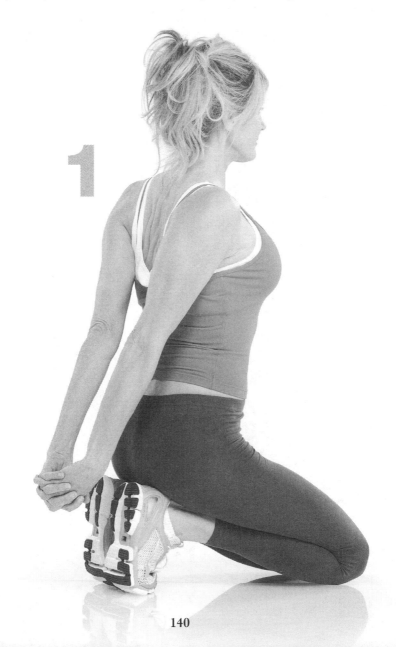

Stretching

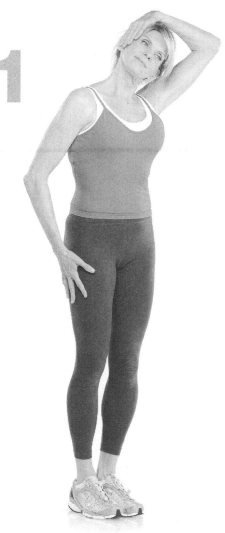

Neck Stretch

Move: Sit or stand tall. Press your shoulders down by pulling your shoulder blades down deep into your back. Drop your right ear toward your right shoulder. Intensify the stretch by reaching the left arm down and behind or by using your right arm to gently pull your head farther to the right. You should feel this stretch from the area behind the left ear to the tip of the left shoulder. Repeat, dropping the left ear toward the left shoulder. Hold each side for 20 to 30 seconds.

Tips:

- Press your shoulder blades down deep into your back to get your shoulders down and stretch your neck long.
- The stretch can also be performed in rotation. Anchor the shoulder blades and shoulders down deep into your back. Turn your head rather than tipping it.

Stretching

Downward Dog

Move: Kneel on your hands and knees with your hands slightly forward of your shoulders. Have your knees and feet hip distance apart. Lift your hips up into an inverted "V" position with your heels lifted. Press through the hands, opening the shoulders. Bend your knees, bringing your ribs closer to your thighs. Lift your sitting bones high, feeling the lower back moving into an inward curve. Slowly start to straighten the knees. Press your heels toward the floor. Your heels may remain lifted until you gain the flexibility to press them all the way down. Continue to press through the hands, working into the shoulder stretch; lifting the hips to increase the stretch in the hamstring muscles; and pressing the heels down, working into the calf stretch. Hold the stretch for 30 seconds or more.

Tips:

- If you have tight hamstring muscles, modify the posture by bending the knees and straightening them as far as you can, feeling a gentle tug. Do not overstretch.
- The main stretches are in the muscles of the shoulders, hamstrings, and calves. There are subtle stretches in the chest, mid- and upper back, and arms. As you breathe into the stretch, be in tune with your body. Listen not only to the stretches that talk to you but to those that whisper too.
- When pressing the heels to the floor, keep the feet parallel. Do not turn the feet in or out.

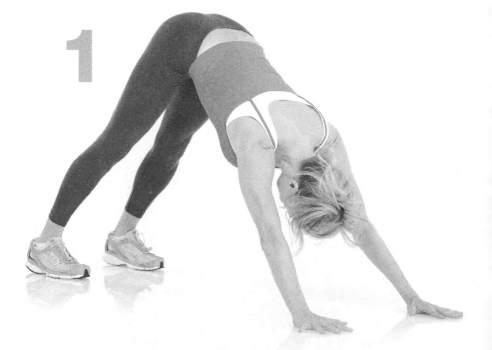

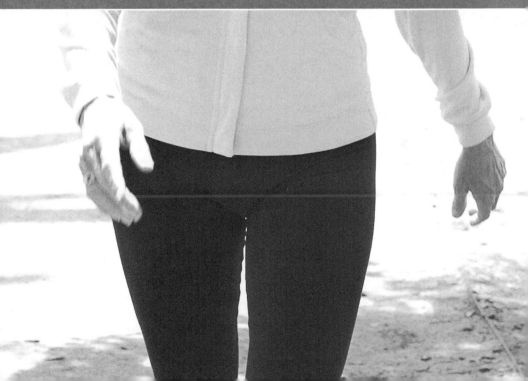

PART 3: THE ART OF LIVING LEAN

You can stay in the best shape of your life for the rest of your life.
It's easy with my Balancing Act and Laws to Living Lean.

Congratulations! Once you reach your target weight, you are ready to enter the last phase of the Feed Muscle, Shrink Fat program—the phase for life. I call it the Balancing Act. You have more than a leaner, fitter body. You are a whole new you with a whole new approach to living.

You've shifted your eating and exercise behaviors, you've changed the way you buy and cook food, you have a realistic understanding about how protein, vitamin C, fiber, fat, and sugar all play a role in your diet, and you've made several deposits into your bank of longevity.

Food is no longer the enemy. It's a source of bountiful energy and youth. You can appreciate the pleasures that come with eating fresh, wholesome foods, and you will never go back to a yo-yo cycle of body chaos. You are prepared to maintain your best shape and healthy eating habits for the rest of your life.

THE BALANCING ACT: BEYOND WEEK 6

The Balancing Act is about staying attuned to your body's needs and desires. It is about knowing when you can let life get in the way momentarily and when you should pull back and pay closer attention to lean proteins and vegetables again.

The Balancing Act is simple: You live within the same basic guidelines of Weeks 3 to 6, but you also have more options so you can enjoy life to its fullest. That doesn't mean you can have a slice of cheesecake every night. It means being mindful of your eating behaviors and body's needs. It means reminding yourself of your trigger foods and knowing the difference between giving yourself permission to have a special treat and fueling an abusive relationship with sugar, fat, and salt. It means having a sensibility about nutrition and living out this newfound sensibility every day as best you can. There are no forbidden foods. There is no "diet" full of restrictions and limits. You have insights now about food and nutrition that will guide you. Listen to your body. It will speak to you when you let it.

Reaching a new fitness level (and waist size) is just the beginning. Now you will maintain this new you—and new lifestyle—with a permanent strategy.

You should remember that there is always an excuse for not exercising or not taking better care of yourself, just as there are always opportunities to eat poorly. We have weddings and parties to attend. We find ourselves away from home without easy access to nutritious meals. We have stressful periods when we have to work long hours and are too low on energy to even think about exercise.

It is all OK. I want you to understand that there is a give and take to maintaining a healthy lifestyle. My weight doesn't stagnate. For 90 percent of the time, I eat within the Feed Muscle, Shrink Fat guidelines. But the other 10 percent of the time, anything goes. I allow myself to have second helpings, I eat out more often than I should, or I indulge in too many desserts. If and when I sense my weight creeping up, I don't let anxiety take control. *I* take control and remind myself that a focus on that Feed Muscle, Shrink Fat equation—protein plus fiber plus vitamin C equals weight loss—will get me back on track in no time. It will help you get back on track too.

When to Repeat Maximum Fat Burn
If you have not arrived at your ideal weight by the end of Week 6, stay at the Maximum Fat Burn stage. I encourage you to be patient with this process.

When to Repeat Fast Track 1
Whenever you feel that you have fallen off the wagon, remind yourself that real success comes from having the strength to pursue your dream of living a healthier lifestyle in a world full of obstacles and excuses. You will find that repeating Fast Track 1 comes in handy if your healthy eating habits have been sidelined. You can do Fast Track for a full week, but you also can build Fast Track days regularly into your life as a way of staying more in tune with your body and its needs. It is often too easy to let an occasional splurge become a regular habit, like eating ice cream several times a week. A quick dip into Fast Track can be your lifeline to a healthier way of living that supports the vision you have for yourself.

I commend and congratulate you on just selecting this book. I hope that with my techniques and ideas, you say goodbye to measuring self-esteem by a number on the scale. I hope that you say hello to rating your success by improvements in relationships, work, family, and productivity. At the end of the day, that is all that really matters. And you are the one in charge.

How Often Should I Weigh Myself?

Don't let the scale run your life. Your body will naturally fluctuate within five pounds, so don't weigh yourself every day. Choose one day a week to check in, such as Friday morning. If your weight is up, don't panic. Focus on lean proteins and vegetables for a few days and the extra pounds will come off. Remember that you can return to Fast Track 1 anytime; it can be especially useful after holidays or before swimsuit season. Think of Fast Track as a safety net. It is the zone you can enter for a reboot whenever necessary.

LAWS TO LIVING LEAN

I have shared with you my diet and fitness secrets to get you in the best shape of your life. But there is one more component to the Feed Muscle, Shrink Fat program that will help you move past potential pitfalls and excuses on your way to a healthier life: my Laws to Living Lean. They can help prevent the days that threaten to derail our efforts and smooth over the times when life gets overly busy. My laws will give you important tools for problem solving. With practice these strategies will become a skill set that will help you make good, healthy decisions day in and day out. You can use these laws for the rest of your life. They will ultimately help you live the Feed Muscle, Shrink Fat way of life for years and years.

LAW NO. 1: Think Progress, Not Perfection

Anything worth accomplishing takes time, patience, and incremental effort, especially when the goal is a profound one. The thought of losing weight can be overwhelming. You are not sure how long the process will take, and you worry that you will not succeed. This is when it is important to think progress, not perfection. Always remember that all the little shifts you make will add up to large changes overall. This process does not happen overnight. Your success will be cumulative.

Last year I climbed Mount Kilimanjaro. The thought of reaching the top was both incredibly motivating and a bit daunting. But no one climbs a mountain in one giant leap. I kept my focus on putting one foot in front of the other. All those little steps add up! As long as you move forward—even by a few inches—you *will* get where you are going eventually.

Think inside out.

And don't forget that as you make slight shifts in your life, a tremendous amount of invisible activity goes on inside your body. Even though you may not see results as quickly as you want on the outside of your body, you are retraining your body's metabolic pathways to more efficiently metabolize food and burn fat. You are changing your body on both a cellular and a hormonal level. Don't beat yourself up if you can't follow the program exactly on a busy day. Focus on the positive: You are exercising most days of the week now and you are eating in a way that is good for your body. One day won't set you back in the grand scheme of things. Remind yourself that you are still moving forward.

Halting Weight Gain

If you suddenly gain weight—and you want to stop it before it spirals out of control—remind yourself of the main tenets of the Feed Muscle, Shrink Fat Diet. To do so ask yourself these questions:

✳ Am I focusing on lean proteins and high-fiber vegetables?

✳ Am I sneaking in too many sugary sweets like candy and soda?

✳ Am I eating too much bread and pasta?

✳ Am I getting at least 30 minutes of exercise a day?

✳ Am I sleeping poorly or experiencing a lot of stress in my life right now?

✳ Am I starving at the beginning of each meal and then overeating because I'm not grazing on snacks in between?

✳ Am I eating in restaurants more and not paying attention to my choices and portions?

✳ Am I overdoing my portions?

✳ Am I oversnacking or eating desserts every night?

✳ Am I letting my family's wants and needs come before my own?

Be honest about your efforts.

If you do not see the results you want, make a bigger commitment to yourself while sticking with the program. Take it seriously and believe in yourself. You *will* see a difference. Don't use "it is not working" as yet another excuse to avoid the journey.

LAW NO. 2: View Exercise as Nonnegotiable

We don't think about whether we will eat, drink, and sleep. We do those things quite robotically because they keep us alive. We can all agree that regular exercise benefits our health and keeps us alive. Yet many of us don't do any exercise. I believe the body emits signals when it is not getting enough exercise, but some of us choose to ignore those signals. When you get into the routine of exercising frequently, you will start to tune in to your body's signals when it is time to get moving and break a sweat. You can get to a place where you are so in sync with your body that those exercise signals become impossible to ignore. They can be very big motivators.

Don't give in to excuses.

To keep up regular daily exercise, be prepared to battle common lifestyle issues. These are some of the excuses I hear most often and ways to move past them:

"I have no time to exercise." Well, who does? Until you make exercise a priority, you won't be able to find time. Consider this: If the president of the United States and executives of top companies can fit in exercise, so can you. (The reason they do is because the investment of time exercising yields benefits at work. They come to the job with more energy and are capable of accomplishing more.) This excuse is particularly hard to use because my workout program can be done in just 10 minutes. I don't know anyone who can't find at least 10 extra minutes a day, if not several pockets of 10 minutes scattered throughout the day. With my Matrix system of moves, you will get a total body workout—working all your muscles in a short period of time. And with the progression of movements through various intensities, you will be amazed at what you can accomplish in just 10 minutes. However, until you understand the value that exercise can bring to your life, you will not carve out time for it.

"I only have a few minutes here and there." Don't fall into the trap of thinking that your workout program has to be completed every day in one continuous segment. All the research indicates that you get the same health benefits by doing three 10-minute bouts of exercise as you would from doing a single 30-minute workout. If you are short on time, go ahead and break up your routine in manageable, bite-size pieces. The Matrix system is designed with this in mind. You can even multitask, watching the morning news as you complete a set of full-body moves that will rev you up for the day. Think of other ways to sneak in more activity during the day and combine socializing and/or work with exercise. For example, break away from your office routine and go with coworkers for a brisk walk.

"I'm too tired to exercise." Try moving your workouts to the morning, when the day's events haven't kicked in to either disrupt you or wear you down. Make sure you are getting enough sleep too (see pages 155–156). Sometimes to get motivated I will make myself a vitamin C drink, then lie on the floor to do inversions where I get my hips above my shoulders so the blood flows to my head. Everyone may need something different to get over that initial hump. But for most everyone the first five minutes are the hardest. Once you get the circulation going and the heart beating faster, the body takes over. It is like the law of inertia: A body in action tends to stay in motion. A little sugar also can be a helpful jumpstart. Try chewing a piece of gum, then take some deep breaths and think about how wonderful you will feel after working out.

"Exercise is boring." This excuse is difficult to understand because there are so many way to mix up exercises with my Matrix system. In Part 2 I discussed the "same time, same place" mentality that takes spontaneity out of exercise. Stop thinking of exercise as drudgery and view it as time for yourself. We all lead stressful, busy lives. Having more time for yourself should be a blessing.

"I didn't get the results I wanted so I gave up." When people say this I question how committed they were to a program and giving their body time to respond. From the moment you start changing how you eat and exercise, your body undergoes a multitude of invisible changes, all of which build a strong foundation for dramatic future results. Remember, we are not aiming just for weight loss. We seek much more: Robust hearts and immune systems. More lean muscle. A strong skeletal system to support other systems and organs. A lower risk for age-related diseases and a slowdown in the degenerative process that affects everything.

LAW NO. 3: Shop Smart at the Grocery Store

Although your grocery shopping habits may change on the Feed Muscle, Shrink Fat program, the store you shop at doesn't need to change. Most local markets today have a wonderful selection of fresh fruits and vegetables, healthy dairy products, lean meats and proteins, legumes, nuts, and seeds. Once you start my meal plan and introduce your body to delicious, wholesome foods, it will be easier to hit those checkout lines without picking up impulse items that are full of excess fat, sugar, and salt. Just follow these tips for navigating the store:

Stick to the perimeter.
Most markets have a similar layout. Meats, produce, and dairy are found around the perimeter, with processed foods (the most concentrated area of junk "goodies" and convenience foods full of unnecessary fats, sugars, carbs, and salt) in the center. When you stay on the perimeter, you stick "close to the earth," buying foods closest to their natural state. You will, however, have to hunt down the grains aisle, which is probably somewhere in the middle.

Shop at the same store.
Once you are accustomed to the store layout at one location, you can shop more efficiently. Avoid the aisles with temptations and save time.

Bring a list.
Avoid buying items not on your list. Don't buy the foods that tempt you to overeat or they will be lurking around at home when your next late-night craving strikes. If you have to buy treats for others in your family, store them deep in the pantry where they are out of sight.

Don't shop when you are hungry.
Do your best to go to the grocery store on a full stomach. You know what happens when you shop hungry. Everything looks good, and you arrive home with bags of extra food, much of it falling in the sugary/salty/fatty category.

Read labels.
It is no surprise that one way to support healthy weight loss is to be conscious about what we buy in the grocery store by reading labels. This is true even for "healthy" products that are labeled "fat-free," "lite," and "low-fat." You may be surprised to see that they include unhealthy ingredients that can sabotage even the most conscientious eater. Ingredients are listed on labels in order from highest content to lowest. If, for example, sugar is the first ingredient listed, that product contains high amounts of sugar as compared with other ingredients.

Kathy's Secret: You can download and print handy grocery lists from my website, kathysmith.com. Take them with you the next time you go grocery shopping.

If taking the time to read labels during a busy shopping trip seems like too much of a hassle, plan to visit the store just to read labels. Think of it as a timesaving exploration that will set you up for success on future shopping trips. Jot down a list of the brands and items you find that are both healthy and delicious. Add those items to your shopping list each week and you will be able to grab them and keep the cart rolling. Or practice label reading with items you already have at home. It won't take long before you read labels out of habit.

Embrace fresh and frozen veggies.
I encourage you to select fresh produce when it is in season. Nothing beats the crunch of a fresh red bell pepper or the sweetness of fresh blueberries. However, certain fresh vegetables can be hard to find depending on the season, and some fresh vegetables are expensive. If you opt for frozen varieties, be assured that because they are frozen immediately after harvest, the nutritional values are about the same as fresh produce.

Buy canned foods.
Canned goods like beans, legumes, and tomatoes are also nutritionally sound alternatives to fresh produce. Watch the sodium content, however, and always go for fresh produce if possible.

Talk to the butcher.

Ask the butcher which meats and fish are the best that day and choose fresh, fresh, fresh. If you find a beautiful cut of steak, you won't have to fuss much with seasoning. A shake of salt, pepper, and maybe some garlic powder and you are minutes away from dinner. The same goes for fish. If the market just received trout fillets, brush them with some olive oil, lay them on a grill pan, add sliced veggies, and you can have dinner in no time.

Find timesavers.

In a hurry? Head to the deli for delicious, healthy prepared foods such as whole roasted chickens or poached fish. Just be sure to avoid fatty sauces and preparations. No time to clean and chop veggies? Take advantage of packaged precut produce or visit the salad bar to buy it by the pound. Canned proteins, like tuna or salmon packed in water also are good to keep on hand for quick salads and sandwiches. Be sure to drain them well.

LAW NO. 4: Make Your Home a Healthy Environment

Your environment should support your healthy eating habits. Create positive energy in your kitchen with how you stock and organize it, just as you create a certain energy in your home with your choice and placement of furniture. Do an inventory of your kitchen, then do the following:

- Discard anything that contains trans fats, hydrogenated fats, high-fructose corn syrup, or added sugars.
- Replace high-fructose corn syrup-based condiments, spreads, and salad dressings with natural, organic alternatives.
- Discard items with artificial sweeteners made with chemicals. (Splenda® and stevia are OK to keep if you must use sweetener.)
- Place any family treats, such as cookies and after-school snacks, far from view. Don't have a cookie jar out on the counter unless you fill it with something like whole fruit or whole grain pasta.
- Replace sugary beverages (including fruit juices and sodas) with still or sparkling water. Have them visible and available when you open the refrigerator. Drink up all day long!
- Replace lard, butter, and margarine with extra virgin olive oil, canola oil, and nut-based oils, plus a cooking spray.
- Dump chips, crackers (except whole grain), cookies, ice cream, candy, and packaged sweets. Avoid having crunchy, salty chips/crackers, trail mix, pretzels, kettle corn, chocolate, and packaged snacks around to tempt you.

- Replace regular mayonnaise with a reduced fat, fat-free, soy- or canola-based mayonnaise.
- Replace full-fat cheeses with lower-fat cheeses.

LAW NO. 5: Consider Your Past Habits

You are sitting on the couch with your kids watching television when a bag of salted chips comes your way. You ask yourself, should I have one? You know that each chip is only about 10 calories, and that isn't much. This is when you need to recall previous times you were in the same situation. Did you eat just one? If you didn't—and you ate half a bag, which is 600 calories—then the best decision today is to pass the bag to someone else.

I advise anyone who is trying to lose weight (and keep it off) to identify her own eating patterns. Tune in to the foods and eating situations that often trigger overeating or binges. Everyone is different when it comes to trigger foods. I used to have a problem with chocolate. If it was in my kitchen it didn't last long. One bite led to two, then three and four. At one point I banished it from my house because there was no chance I could eat it in moderation. I have learned that it is usually easier to simply say "no" to even one chip or candy. It is much harder to stop a binge when it is in progress.

Kathy's Secret: Every choice you make today—whether to buy strawberries or brownies—is your decision. All those small choices you make determine whether you step closer or farther from the body that you want.

Rely on your journal.

Our bodies and our fitness levels are created by old habits and old patterns. That is why keeping a journal is so helpful. (See pages 81 and 82 for journal page samples.) It is just as important to write about your feelings as it is to record what you eat and which exercises you do. Keeping notes helps you become more aware of your habits and patterns, and with that awareness you can learn how to shift them in a healthier direction. It is like missing the forest for the trees: In the hum of daily life, we're often unaware of how our behavior falls into patterns and how we repeat the same mistakes until we see it recorded on paper.

In reviewing my own journal, for instance, I discovered that I have a habit of eating trail mix right from the bag. That can lead me to eat multiple servings. I didn't realize until I did the math how many calories I was mindlessly consuming. Now I remind myself to measure out one portion so I don't overeat. Watch your journal to see which habits you need to break.

Ban It! The High-Fructose Corn Syrup Danger

I want you to ban high-fructose corn syrup (HFCS) immediately from your kitchen and your diet. This will have a major impact on your health and ability to lose weight. HFCS is a highly processed sugar with no nutritional value. It is a cheap ingredient that food manufacturers use to make products taste better and extend their shelf life. HFCS packs more calories into food and beverages than most people realize. Recent studies point to a link between the rapid rise in obesity and HFCS, which has been used since the 1970s. HFCS also affects the balance of your body's digestive hormones. When you consume HFCS your brain never gets the "I'm full, stop eating" message, so imagine what this means for your waistline! The good news is that there are always healthy alternatives to HFCS foods. (Note: Fructose, which is the main ingredient in HFCS, is not the same as the major component in regular white table sugar, or sucrose. It is also different from glucose, which is the main source of fuel for the body and especially the brain.)

You will find HFCS in all kinds of processed and sweetened products, including cereals, sodas, salad dressings, condiments (ketchup, creamy mustards), ice cream, and some yogurts. It also is found in many products labeled "fat-free," "lite," or "low-fat." That is because the manufacturers remove the fat and replace it with diet-unfriendly HFCS. Remember, as part of a balanced diet fat can be good for you because it helps you feel full sooner.

LAW NO. 6: Seek Substitutions for What You Crave

It is unrealistic to think you won't be tempted to overindulge in your favorite sugary, salty, or fatty snack foods while on the Feed Muscle, Shrink Fat program. But you can be prepared by having healthy substitutions available. Replace addictive foods with other options. Sometimes it is simply a certain texture that we seek. If you love crunchy chips with ranch dressing, try crunchy celery or sweet peppers with hummus or an all-natural, low-fat dressing. If you are in the mood for candy, try fruit with a little protein and healthy fat for satiety. A berry-based smoothie with a drop of flaxseed oil may do the trick. My snack list (page 43) offers dozens of ideas.

Follow the 10 percent rule.

Once you reach your goal weight, don't completely deprive yourself. If you can find healthier substitutes for your cravings 90 percent of the time, feel free to indulge in your favorite foods the other 10 percent of the time. The truth is that no food is totally bad. It is all in how much you eat. I eat chocolate occasionally, but I prefer to have it when I'm away from home. I don't keep it in my kitchen because that is too much temptation. When you reach your ideal weight, part of maintaining your new body will entail knowing when to allow yourself a small portion of a favorite food and when you should seek a substitution instead. This program will get you attuned to your body in a way that makes this decision easy.

LAW NO. 7: Detach Mood from Food

Sometimes when you have had a really bad/stressful/exhausting/boring day, you arrive home and all you want to eat is a pint of ice cream and a bag of barbecue potato chips. Sound familiar? Sometimes eating is not about hunger. Mood eating is one of the most overwhelming issues for any weight-conscious person. We often turn to comfort foods for reasons other than fuel, and distinguishing the physical need from the emotional need—especially in the heat of the moment—can be one of the hardest things to do. Boredom, loneliness, anger, sadness, anxiety, frustration, and fatigue are all controlling emotions. The key is to strike a balance between knowing what you eat and understanding how you feel.

Pour your feelings into a journal.

This is when keeping a journal becomes critical. I have led many groups through weight loss programs, and I account much of their success to their dedication in keeping food-mood entries. Everyone recorded how they felt before and after they ate. You will do this on my program as well. Take time to write what you feel the moment you sense that you want to head to the kitchen for some out-of-control eating. Are you tired, lonely, bored, upset? Which emotion is taking over? Does this emotion connect with a particular food or need for a particular taste sensation? Are you truly hungry or just looking for a way to deal with the emotion?

Especially if you are an emotional eater (see page 18), write about how life is affecting your eating habits and include notes on the days you veer off track and respond to being angry, lonely, bored, or tired with food.

This will help you come to a better understanding of your personal connection between mood and food. As you continue to fill your journal, you will gain self-awareness to help you make better decisions when the same mood pattern repeats. The goal is to reach a point where you no longer eat in response to negative feelings. If you find, for example, that you become cranky around 4:30 every afternoon and you munch on something that you later regret, you may want to plan a 20-minute walk at that time and have a light snack ready when you return.

LAW NO. 8: Think Quality of Calories, Not Number

Let's face it, counting calories or grams of this and that is impractical. It is not very useful when trying to lose weight because, as Part 1 teaches you, not all calories are created equal. A 300-calorie candy bar is not equivalent to a 300-calorie turkey wrap. Your body responds differently to these foods. The sugary candy bar is likely to feed your fat cells, whereas the high-protein wrap will feed muscle, fostering a chain of events that results in a higher metabolism, preserved lean muscle mass, and blood sugar balance. By following my Feed Muscle, Shrink Fat program, you will learn to distinguish between fat bombs that enlarge fat cells and the nutrient goodies (lean proteins, fibrous fruits and vegetables, healthy fats, and whole grains) that keep you constantly nourished and healthy.

LAW NO. 9: Remember the Power of R&R ... and Your Zzz's

Most of us know that constant stress is not good for our health. Neither is sleep deprivation, which is linked to everything from an increased risk of hypertension, diabetes, and obesity to an elevated risk for depression, heart attack, and stroke.

Make sleep a priority.

A good night's sleep now appears to be every bit as important to good health and long life as a nutritious diet and regular exercise. In 2004 researchers showed a strong connection between sleep and the ability to lose weight. The more you sleep the better your body can regulate the hormones that control hunger and appetite. Two digestive hormones—ghrelin and leptin—work together to control your feelings of hunger and appetite. Your stomach secretes ghrelin when it is empty, telling your brain that you are hungry and increasing your appetite. When you are full, leptin sends your brain the opposite message so you quit eating.

Inadequate sleep creates an imbalance of both ghrelin and leptin, thus impeding your brain's ability to get the message that you are full. So you keep eating and eating. One study at the University of Chicago showed that when people were allowed just four hours of sleep a night for two nights, they suffered a 20 percent drop in leptin and an increase in ghrelin. They also had a 24 percent increase in hunger and a 23 percent increase in appetite. Their appetite for calorie-dense, high-carbohydrate foods like sweets, salty snacks, and starchy foods increased by 33 to 45 percent.

The lesson: Don't underestimate the power of sleep. Sleep has other benefits as well, such as supporting a healthy immune system, keeping you energetic, and helping your memory stay sharp. Growth hormone is largely secreted during the night in deep sleep. In addition to helping cells repair and renew themselves, growth hormone helps control the body's ratio of fat to muscle. Sleep also plays a major role in how well we age and how healthy we "look" (think about skin repair and rejuvenation). The ever-beating heart needs sleep too. During the night the heart gets a break.

We all have a bad night's sleep from time to time. When you do, take extra care of yourself the next day. Instead of reaching for sugary or fatty snacks, focus on lean proteins like fish, turkey, or eggs that will keep you satisfied until your next meal. Then take some time that evening to slow down and relax to ensure a better night's sleep.

Focus on relaxation.

Stress is the enemy of achievement. It disrupts the body and clouds the mind. Stress causes a cascade of problems, all of which lead to a state of unhealthiness and a poor sense of well-being. In fact stress can be so disruptive of the overall balance and immune function of the body that it can ultimately cause some forms of cancer. When your body is stressed, which happens when we feel tired and overworked, it will trip an increase in the production of the hormones cortisol and adrenaline, which can lead to intense cravings. This causes your body to hold tightly to fat, leading to weight gain. The key is to limit stress and adopt healthy methods for coping with the rigors of daily life.

Need help relaxing? You will find lots of ideas and products to help calm and focus your mind on kathysmith.com. Some people read a book or take a warm bath. Exercise can be a terrific form of relaxation. Others enjoy meditation, which may slow the aging-related atrophy of certain areas of the brain. In other words, meditation not only helps you better cope with stress but also may help you keep your brain young and functioning optimally. Experiment with new techniques to see what works best for you. One trick I use is simply to take a few deep belly

Kathy's Secret: Breathing exercises can decrease stress and improve mental and physical health. Find more ideas on how to unwind and relax at kathysmith.com. You also can write to me about your personal experiences with the Feed Muscle, Shrink Fat program. Share your own tips and ask questions on an active message board. I will post the most frequently asked questions and give great solutions. Your questions will contribute to an active guide!

breaths. Here is how you do it:

- Place your hands along your rib cage at the level of your sternum.
- As you inhale you should feel your belly and rib cage expand.
- Exhale and feel your belly and rib cage collapse.
- Take four to six long breaths, inhaling for six counts, exhaling for six counts.
- Do this a few times a day.

You soon will notice a shift in your attitude, and your stress level may lower.

LAW NO. 10: Start Every Day with Breakfast

When you eat is as important as what you eat. This is a point I stress repeatedly, and it starts with breakfast. You should eat breakfast within one hour of rising. It can work wonders on your body's metabolism and overall ability to lose weight and keep it off.

Although you probably have heard this advice before, you may not know why it is such a great idea. After seven to eight hours of sleep, eating breakfast is like flipping a magical switch that turns on your metabolism and sets the stage for your blood sugar, energy level, and even your mood for that day. Skipping breakfast is proven to make weight control more difficult. People who skip a morning meal eat more food at the next meal, eat high-calorie snacks to curb hunger, struggle to fight off low energy and sleepiness in the late afternoon, and have a hard time fitting important nutrients into their diet.

Here is something else to keep in mind: Your brain runs on glucose—the fuel you need to think, walk, talk, and carry on virtually all activities. If you skip breakfast,0it becomes much harder to accomplish things, including exercise. When you go a long time without fuel, your body responds naturally by entering a "safe mode" and slowing down its metabolism. When you do eventually eat, chances are you are going to overeat. The human body accumulates more fat when you eat fewer, larger meals, so you are better off eating breakfast even if you don't feel hungry.

The lesson: Commit to eating a wholesome breakfast. Eating breakfast has been proved (many times) to not only stimulate metabolism and help with weight and cholesterol control but also to improve concentration, problem-solving ability, mental performance, memory, and mood. By eating breakfast you set yourself up for maintaining healthy eating habits throughout the day.

Breakfast bests.

What you choose to eat will set the tone for the entire day. And there's no excuse for breaking my "eat breakfast every day" rule when there are such deliciously healthy options. Here are some ideas and guidelines for choosing hearty breakfast foods that are high in protein and fiber.

Cereals: Select a high-fiber, whole grain variety that is also low in sugar. It can be hot or cold. High-fiber means it delivers at least 4 or 5 grams per 100 calories; "low in sugar" means it contains no more than 5 grams total.

Add fat-free, soy-based, or low-fat milk and top with antioxidant-rich berries like blueberries or raspberries. Make hot cereals, such as old-fashioned or steel-cut oats, with fat-free or low-fat milk or water. Add a tablespoon of ground flax-seed for omega-3s and extra fiber, plus a dash of cinnamon for flavor and you have a heart-healthy breakfast. For a touch of sweetness, add a teaspoon of agave nectar or a pinch of natural brown sugar. Top with 3 to 5 crushed raw walnuts and berries.

Eggs: Eggs get a standing ovation. Packed with high-quality protein, B vitamins, and the antioxidant selenium, eggs are one of the world's perfect foods. They do contain a small amount of saturated fat (about 1.5 grams) and cholesterol, but they still deliver a wholesome punch of nutrients. You can eliminate some fat and cholesterol by mixing whole eggs with egg whites (see "Living Lean Summary," page 75). Try two egg whites with salsa or sliced tomatoes on a piece of whole grain toast with salt and pepper to taste. Wash it all down with a glass of fat-free, low-fat, or soy-based milk. Enjoy all the herbs and spices you want. Chopped fresh cilantro or parsley and a sprinkle of light Parmesan cheese can turn plain eggs into a delightful meal with intense flavor.

Waffles, pancakes, muffins: These tend to be the heavyweights at the breakfast table, high in calories and saturated fat and low in nutrients. See if you can switch to healthier varieties by turning to whole grain versions that contain fiber. Watch portion sizes. Instead of dousing pancakes and waffles with syrup made mostly with corn syrup, opt for the real thing—100 percent pure maple syrup. Use just a small drizzle. If you are insulin resistant or diabetic, try agave nectar. You can see from my recipes like the Lemon Ricotta Pancakes and Quick-Fix Waffle Breakfast that I choose high-quality ingredients and increase the amount of protein and vitamins without sacrificing flavor.

Yogurt, fruit, nuts: Nothing could be easier than a cup of plain fat-free yogurt mixed with berries and a few crushed nuts. For more volume and a dose of healthy fat, add a spoonful of ground flaxseed.

LAW NO. 11: Eat Every Three to Four Hours

You should eat every three to four hours. Eating smaller meals during the day with snacks will keep you satisfied, increase your metabolic rate, preserve lean muscle mass, and keep your moods consistent. If you go too long without eating, you can actually cause your body to hold on to fat (to protect itself) and consume muscle. This then translates to burning fewer calories and feeling low on energy.

The proof is in the research. Scandinavian scientists recently tested two diets with a group of athletes who were trying to lose weight. Although all of them lost the same amount of weight, those who ate more frequent meals lost almost all *fat* tissue. At Nagoya University in Japan athletes who ate six meals a day preserved their muscle tissue as they lost weight, whereas the ones who ate the same number of calories in just two daily meals *lost* muscle tissue.

LAW NO. 12: Think Big

We are all sidetracked once in a while. That is OK. We become frustrated by the little stuff—like five extra pounds or a pair of pants that don't fit—and forget to consider the larger picture. Stay focused and remember the vision you have for yourself. When we move from having a constant microscope on our ourselves to appreciating a more macrocosmic perspective, we can usher in a passionate attitude that has the effect of weakening the fixation on food.

Head out on a Gratitude Walk.

In the last several years I have started to take what I call Gratitude Walks. I step outside my home and go on a mindful walk, taking in the details of my surroundings: The curvature of the trees. The individual petals of blooming flowers. The color of the sky and the shapes of the clouds. These are details we rarely appreciate in daily living. The walks make me aware and vigilant, and I become exceptionally thankful for my life and the world in which I live.

When you are present in the moment like this, you start to think in a whole new light and connect in ways you never imagined. You also become inspired, thinking more broadly rather than focusing on your own inner world and trivial frustrations. Suddenly you are motivated to take on something bigger than yourself—like a charity walk or 10K. You find that participating in life fills you to the point where food truly becomes something that nourishes and sustains you. It doesn't have to be an obsession all the time. You don't have to give up your job, join the Peace Corps, or go to any great lengths to "think big." Just take note of what goes on in your own community and be involved. I bet you will be surprised by how it can change you.

LAW NO. 13: You Can Tame Your Sugar Habit

Almost all of us love something sweet, whether it is a piece of chocolate or a slice of fruit pie. So on the Feed Muscle, Shrink Fat program, you don't have to nix sugar entirely. But I do recommend that in the beginning of this program you

Weight Loss Secrets and Science

In 1994 doctors established the National Weight Control Registry (NWCR), which meticulously tracks about 6,000 people who have lost more than 30 pounds and kept it off. The registry is the largest prospective investigation of long-term successful weight loss maintenance, and some of its findings are remarkable:

* Long-term weight losers eat breakfast no matter what and step on the scale about once a week to "check in." They also keep food diaries, which allow them to respond quickly to changes in their eating patterns. The Feed Muscle, Shrink Fat plan salutes these smart ideas.

* Those who maintain weight loss for two to five years cut in half their risk of regaining the weight.

* Even though about half the people in the registry were overweight as children and three-quarters had at least one parent who was overweight, they were still able to lose the pounds. This is good news for people who falsely believe they "can't" lose weight because it is "in their genes."

severely restrict it for a few days or, if you can, a week. This will help you release your craving and recalibrate your blood sugar.

It is all about understanding how different foods affect your body so you can make informed choices about how and when to eat sweets. Sweets don't have to be taboo if you learn to manage them so that the occasional indulgence doesn't get in the way of fitness goals. Sugar is unique in that it can fuel cravings and throw a blood sugar level so out of whack that it becomes nearly impossible to control your portions. The key is to know which foods and sugar-laden products you can handle and which ones you should eliminate from your kitchen entirely.

Start by noticing how sugar affects you. Identify which foods you absolutely cannot control. We all know people who can eat a few M&M's® and walk away, while other people end up eating the whole bag. Sugar affects these people in very different ways. If you have something sweet, do you instantly crave more? Do you feel lethargic or tired? Do you feel mentally foggy or unwell in general? If so, you probably don't process sugar very well. You need to respect your body's reaction to sugar and find a new way of enjoying sweets without making yourself sick. Reducing your sugar habit probably won't eliminate its effect on you when you have it, but it will make it easier to say "no thanks" more often.

To maintain your sugar sanity, try these tricks:

Don't eat sugar when you are hungry. A sugary snack on an empty stomach is more likely to trigger a craving, causing you to eat far more of the sweet treat than you would if you were full.

Eat a sweet after a meal. You are less likely to eat a lot of a sweet after a balanced meal. Make sure you have had a good source of protein in your meal (such as grilled salmon or halibut, lean beef, chicken, or turkey). The protein diminishes the impact of the sugar on your system.

Prep for dessert. If you sit down to a meal and you know that you will want dessert, make sure to eliminate starchy carbohydrates from that meal, including bread, pasta, and grains. Your dessert will count as a starch.

Eat sweets very slowly. Savor the taste and texture. Set down your fork or spoon between bites. When you really enjoy what you eat, you won't need a huge amount to satisfy your craving.

Be discriminating. Once you start savoring your sweets, you will notice the quality of what you are eating. Put down the inferior chocolate and tell yourself it is just not good enough for your taste buds. You don't want to waste calories on anything inferior.

Let go of the guilt. Guilt is not a good weight loss motivator—it can actually make you eat more, not less. When you think of sweets as a no-no, you feel you have to sneak them. Sneaking often leads to gobbling and making poor choices about what to have. Change your relationship to sweets so that you control them instead of letting them control you.

Be prepared. Handle your cravings by anticipating them. If you know that you react to sugar by craving more (and more), have a plan ready to help your body metabolize the sugar. Effective tools include doing something else that feels good to take your mind off the urge, such as taking a relaxing bath.

LAW NO. 14: You Can Eat at Restaurants

It is true that many restaurants serve portions that are enough for a small family. The same amount of pasta served to a 120-pound woman also is served to a 250-pound man. What is more, restaurant portions typically include only small amounts of protein and limited produce while the refined or starchy carbohydrates are off the charts. On the Feed Muscle, Shrink Fat program, you can still enjoy a night out. Here's how:

Watch protein portions. One serving size of protein is about the size of your palm. If the amount of protein in your entrée is too small, boost it by ordering an appetizer that has a good source of protein or by requesting extra meat, chicken, or tofu on your salad or sandwich. If there is too much protein, ask to take half of your meal home. Doggie bag, please!

Think vegetables first. Request more steamed vegetables, grilled asparagus, or a side salad. If you have a meal that includes a starch, such as bread, rice, or pasta, think about what you really want and watch serving sizes. If you decide on grilled fish and steamed veggies, and you know the bread is fabulous, eat it! But if you decide on a baked potato or rice, you already have your starch and should do without the bread this time.

Be prepared. You have to become mentally prepared for eating out whether it is at a restaurant or at your best friend's house. Eat a mini meal before you head out the door. Be sure to include a good source of lean protein and some fibrous vegetables. Try two hard-cooked eggs with a side of steamed spinach. It will fill your stomach, keep your blood sugar level happy for a while, and stave off hunger and cravings.

Don't be afraid of buffets. Just because it is a buffet doesn't mean you have to go through 10 plates. Stick to serving yourself one plate in line with the Feed Muscle, Shrink Fat plan. If you want to enjoy numerous trips to the tables like everyone else, start with a plate of lean protein (sliced turkey, red meat, or fish), then return for a new plate heavy on fresh steamed vegetables. Leave the starchier carbohydrates, fruits, and sweets for last.

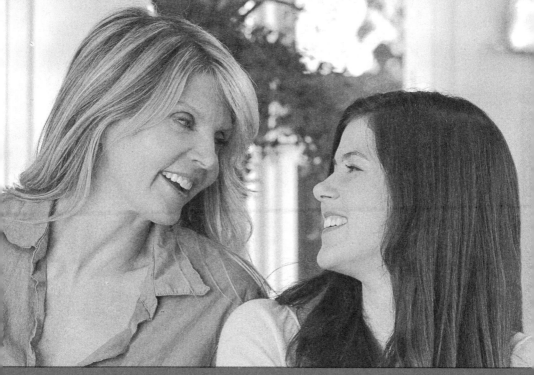

PART 4: THE RECIPES

Whether you're eating at home or at a restaurant, the entire eating experience should be enjoyable. The Feed Muscle, Shrink Fat Diet plan and recipes give you the flexibility needed to live and eat in the real world. Enjoy!

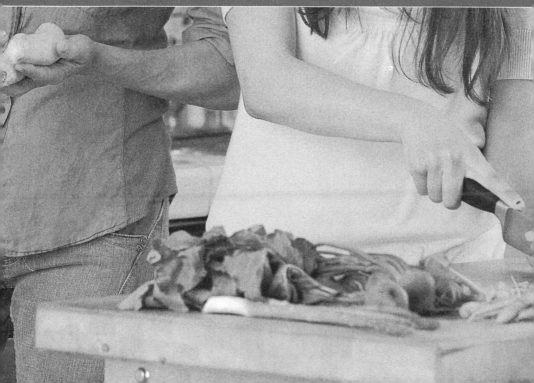

Banana Crisp Yogurt Sundae

1 6-ounce container fat-free plain yogurt
1 small banana, sliced
¼ cup Kashi GoLean® cereal
¼ teaspoon cinnamon

Mix the yogurt with the banana in a small bowl. Top with the cereal and sprinkle with the cinnamon. Serves 1.

Protein Power Sundae

1 6-ounce container fat-free vanilla yogurt
1 tablespoon flaxseed
1 tablespoon vanilla protein powder (such as Jay Robb™ egg white protein powder)
¼ cup blueberries or other fruit

Mix all ingredients together in a small bowl. Serves 1.

Hawaiian Crunch

1   **cup low-fat cottage cheese**
½   **cup cubed fresh pineapple or drained canned pineapple chunks (juice pack)**
½   **cup Kashi GoLean® cereal**

Place cottage cheese in a bowl. Top with pineapple and sprinkle with the cereal. Serves 1.

Kathy's Yogurt Sundae

1   **6-ounce container low-fat blueberry yogurt (all natural, if available)**
¼   **cup raw walnut pieces**
½   **cup sliced strawberries**

Combine all the ingredients in a bowl. Serves 1.

Gazpacho Sundae

4 cucumber slices
4 bell pepper strips
1 cup low-fat cottage cheese
2 to 4 tablespoons fat-free salsa
    Bottled hot pepper sauce (optional)

Arrange cucumber and bell pepper on a plate. Top with cottage cheese and salsa. Add a shake of bottled hot pepper sauce, if desired. Serves 1.

Master Recipe for Steel-Cut Oatmeal

4 cups water
1 cup steel-cut oats

Pour the water into a medium saucepan; bring to boiling. Stir in oats and immediately reduce the heat to low. Cover and simmer for 30 minutes, stirring occasionally. Serve hot. Serves 4.

Note: Leftover oatmeal can be stored in the refrigerator and reheated in the microwave without diminishing the nutty texture.

Master Recipe for Rolled (Old-Fashioned) Oatmeal

3½   cups water
2   cups rolled (old-fashioned) oats

To cook on the stovetop:
Pour water into a medium saucepan; bring to boiling. Stir in oats and immediately reduce to low. Simmer for 3 to 5 minutes, stirring occasionally. Serve hot.

To cook in the microwave:
Combine water and oats in a microwave-safe 2-quart bowl. Microwave on high (100 percent power) for 2 to 4 minutes, depending on the power of the microwave. Take care; the bowl may be very hot! Serve hot. Serves 4.

Note: To reduce the glycemic response, add 1 tablespoon protein powder to either steel-cut or rolled oatmeal, then cook as directed. If you like, add ½ cup soymilk or fat-free milk to the cooked oatmeal for desired texture.

Berry-Oatmeal Crunch

½ **cup hot cooked oatmeal**
½ **cup fresh berries of choice**
¼ **cup chopped toasted almonds**
1 **teaspoon grated orange or lemon zest**

Place oatmeal in a cereal bowl. Stir berries, nuts, and zest into hot oatmeal, taking care not to completely break up the berries. Serve hot. Serves 1.

Cranberry-Oatmeal Crunch

½ **cup hot cooked oatmeal**
⅓ **cup dried cranberries, raisins, or chopped dried figs**
¼ **cup chopped toasted walnuts**
⅛ **teaspoon cinnamon**

Place oatmeal in a cereal bowl. Stir cranberries, walnuts, and cinnamon into hot oatmeal. Serve hot. Serves 1.

Little Figgy Overnight Oatmeal

1   cup steel-cut oats or Kashi® oatmeal
1   cup dried figs, chopped
4   cups water

Mix all ingredients in a slow cooker. Cover and cook on low heat setting for 8 hours. Serves 4.

Quick-Fix Cereals

For hot cereal you'll need:
1   packet instant Irish oatmeal, Kashi® oatmeal, or Cream of Wheat®

Make cereal according to package directions. Serves 1.

Add:
1   to 2 tablespoons vanilla protein powder and 1 teaspoon peanut butter or ¼ cup walnut or almond pieces

For ready-to-eat cereal you'll need:
Kashi GoLean®
Barbara's Bakery® Multigrain Shredded Spoonfuls
Whole Grain Total®
Wheaties®
Product 19®
All-Bran®
Uncle Sam®

Measure out no more than 1 cup of cereal (choose from list above) into a bowl. Add ½ cup fat-free milk or low-fat soymilk. Serves 1.

Lemon Ricotta Pancakes

Berry Compote (recipe follows)
1 **cup rolled (old-fashioned) oats**
8 **egg whites or 1 cup purchased egg whites**
½ **cup ricotta cheese**
1 **teaspoon lemon extract**
1 **tablespoon grated lemon zest**
Nonstick canola oil cooking spray

Prepare Berry Compote; let stand while making pancakes. Combine oats, egg whites, ricotta cheese, lemon extract, and lemon zest in a blender. Cover and blend until smooth.

Mist a nonstick skillet or griddle with nonstick cooking spray. Heat skillet over medium heat for 2 minutes. Cook 2 to 3 large pancakes (one at a time if using a small skillet) until large bubbles appear on the surface. Turn pancakes and continue cooking until browned. Top with Berry Compote. Serves 2 to 3.

Berry Compote

2 **cups mixed fresh berries or frozen berries, thawed**
2 **tablespoons fresh lemon juice**

Mix berries with lemon juice in a bowl. Let stand while making pancakes. For a syrupy consistency, mash berries with a fork. Serves 2 to 3.

Apple-Cinnamon Pancakes

  1 **cup rolled (old-fashioned) oats**
  8 **egg whites or 1 cup purchased egg whites**
$\frac{1}{2}$ **cup low-fat (2 percent) cottage cheese**
$1\frac{1}{2}$ **teaspoons vanilla extract**
$\frac{1}{2}$ **teaspoon ground cinnamon**
    Nonstick canola oil cooking spray
    Poached Cinnamon Apples (recipe follows) or $\frac{1}{2}$ cup no-sugar-added
    applesauce
    Ground cinnamon (optional)

Combine oats, egg whites, cottage cheese, vanilla, and the $\frac{1}{2}$ teaspoon
cinnamon in a blender. Cover and blend until smooth. Mist a nonstick skillet
or griddle with nonstick cooking spray. Heat skillet over medium heat for
2 minutes. Cook 2 to 3 large pancakes (one at a time if using a small skillet)
until large bubbles appear on the surface. Turn pancakes and continue cooking
until browned. Top with Poached Cinnamon Apples or applesauce. Sprinkle
with additional cinnamon, if desired. Serves 2 to 3.

Poached Cinnamon Apples

  2 **sweet apples (such as McIntosh or Golden Delicious), peeled, cored,**
    and chopped
$\frac{1}{2}$ **cup no-sugar-added applesauce**
$\frac{1}{4}$ **teaspoon ground cinnamon**

Heat apples and applesauce in a small saucepan. Cook over medium heat until
apples are tender but not mushy (3 to 5 minutes). Sprinkle with cinnamon; stir
to combine. Serves 2 to 3.

Bananas Foster French Toast

1 whole egg plus 2 egg whites
½ teaspoon vanilla extract
⅛ teaspoon nutmeg
2 slices low-carb wheat bread (such as Rudi's Organic Bakery® Right Choice
   or Oroweat® light bread)
   Nonstick canola oil cooking spray
   Bananas Foster Topping (recipe follows)

Beat eggs, vanilla, and nutmeg in a shallow dish. Place bread slices in egg
mixture; turn to coat and let soak for several minutes or until most of the egg
mixture is absorbed. Mist a nonstick skillet or griddle with nonstick cooking
spray. Heat skillet or griddle over medium heat for 2 minutes. Cook French
toast on both sides until brown (2 to 3 minutes per side). Remove from skillet
and spoon Bananas Foster Topping over French toast. Makes 2 slices.

Bananas Foster Topping

1 medium banana, halved lengthwise and cut into 2-inch chunks
3 tablespoons apple juice
1 tablespoon lemon juice
½ teaspoon ground cinnamon

Combine banana, apple juice, lemon juice, and cinnamon in a small saucepan.
Cook until banana is softened and hot but not mushy (3 to 5 minutes). Spoon
over the French toast.

Ricotta Cheese Sandwich

  1 **slice whole grain bread (such as Ezekiel 4:9® or Rudi's Organic Bakery®)**
  ¼ **cup low-fat ricotta cheese**
  ⅓ **cup sliced fresh fruit (pear, apple, peach, or plum) or ¼ cup dried fruit (snipped figs, apricots, or dates)**
      Cinnamon, nutmeg, or lemon zest (optional)

Toast bread and spread with ricotta cheese. Top with fruit. Sprinkle with cinnamon, if desired. Serves 1.

Nanner-Nutter

  2 **slices Oroweat® light bread or 1 slice regular whole wheat bread**
  2 **tablespoons peanut butter**
  ½ **of a banana, sliced**

Toast bread. Spread with peanut butter. Top with banana slices. Serves 1.

Quick-Fix Waffle Breakfast

  1 **Kashi GoLean® frozen waffle**
  ½ **cup low-fat cottage cheese**
  ½ **cup sliced strawberries or other berries**

Toast waffle. Top with cottage cheese and berries. Serves 1.

Sausage Sandwich

1   turkey or veggie sausage patty
    Nonstick canola oil cooking spray
1   whole egg or 3 egg whites
1   whole wheat English muffin
1   1-ounce slice low-fat (2 percent) cheese
1   slice tomato

Microwave sausage patty according to package directions; set aside. Mist a
nonstick skillet with nonstick cooking spray. Heat skillet over medium heat for
2 minutes. Fry the whole egg (or cook the egg whites) to desired doneness.

Meanwhile, toast English muffin. Place sausage patty on bottom half of
muffin. Top with egg, cheese, tomato, and other half of muffin. Serves 1.

Egg Pita Pocket

    Nonstick canola oil cooking spray
2   whole eggs, 4 to 6 egg whites, or ¾ cup egg substitute
1   whole wheat pita bread (such as Ezekiel 4:9® pita with 90 calories), cut
    crosswise in half
    Sliced veggies (such as tomato, cucumber, or bell pepper)

Mist a nonstick skillet with nonstick cooking spray. Heat the skillet over
medium-high heat for 2 minutes. Lightly beat eggs. Cook eggs in hot skillet
until set. Carefully open pockets in pita bread halves and stuff with eggs and
veggie slices. Eat immediately or wrap it up and take it with you! Serves 1.

Breakfast Burrito

1   turkey or veggie breakfast sausage link
    Nonstick canola oil cooking spray
½   of a green bell pepper, chopped
1   whole egg
3   to 6 egg whites
1   8-inch low-fat whole wheat or low-carb tortilla (such as Mission®)
1   ounce grated low-fat (2 percent) cheese

Cook sausage according to package directions; set aside.

Meanwhile, mist a nonstick skillet with nonstick cooking spray. Heat skillet over medium heat for 2 minutes. Saute bell pepper in hot skillet until tender, about 3 minutes.

Lightly beat egg and egg whites; add to skillet. Cook until eggs are set.

Place eggs on tortilla, leaving a border on all sides. Top with the cheese and the sausage link. Roll up burrito style, tucking in the ends as you go. Serves 1.

Wrap-It-Up Egg Scramble

Nonstick canola oil cooking spray
4 to 6 egg whites (or ¾ cup egg substitute or ¾ cup purchased egg whites)
1 6-inch herb and garlic, scallion, or plain whole wheat tortilla (such as La Tortilla Factory®)
¼ cup fat-free refried beans
1 ounce crumbled feta cheese or finely shredded low-fat (2 percent) cheddar or Monterey Jack cheese
Fat-free salsa (optional)

Mist a nonstick skillet with nonstick cooking spray. Heat the skillet over medium-high heat for 2 minutes. Lightly beat egg whites in a small bowl. Cook egg whites in the hot skillet until set. Remove skillet from heat.

Spread the tortilla with the beans and sprinkle with the cheese. Place cooked eggs on one side of tortilla, add salsa (if desired), and roll up. Serves 1.

Italian-Style Scramble

Nonstick olive oil cooking spray
¼ **cup chopped red bell pepper**
1 **cup packed fresh spinach, torn into bite-size pieces**
1 **whole egg plus 3 egg whites (or ¾ cup egg substitute or ¾ cup egg purchased egg whites)**
2 **to 4 fresh basil leaves, torn (optional)**
1 **tablespoon freshly grated Parmesan cheese (optional)**
Freshly ground pepper

Mist a nonstick skillet with nonstick cooking spray. Heat the skillet over medium-high heat for 2 minutes. Saute the bell pepper in hot skillet until tender (2 to 3 minutes). Add spinach to skillet and stir just until wilted.

Lightly beat whole egg and egg whites in a small bowl. Add eggs to the spinach mixture in skillet. Stir with a rubber spatula until eggs are set. Sprinkle with basil and/or Parmesan cheese, if desired. Season to taste with ground pepper. Serves 1.

Note: If you like, add 1 cooked and crumbled turkey sausage link or slice turkey bacon to the beaten eggs.

Mexican-Style Scramble

Nonstick canola oil cooking spray
¼ **cup chopped green bell pepper**
1 **small tomato, chopped**
1 **whole egg plus 3 egg whites (or ¾ cup egg substitute or ¾ cup egg purchased egg whites)**
   Chopped fresh cilantro (optional)
2 **tablespoons crumbled feta cheese (optional)**

Mist a nonstick skillet with nonstick cooking spray. Heat the skillet over medium-high heat for 2 minutes. Saute bell pepper in hot skillet until tender (2 to 3 minutes). Add tomato and cook just until softened (1 minute).

Lightly beat whole egg and egg whites in a small bowl. Add eggs to the vegetable mixture in skillet. Stir with a rubber spatula until eggs are set. Sprinkle with cilantro and/or feta cheese, if desired. Serves 1.

Note: If you like, add 1 cooked and crumbled turkey sausage link or slice turkey bacon to the beaten eggs.

Deli-Style Scramble

Nonstick canola oil cooking spray
2 **tablespoons chopped red onion (optional)**
2 **ounces smoked salmon, diced**
1 **whole egg plus 3 egg whites (or ¾ cup egg substitute or ¾ cup egg purchased egg whites)**
1 **tablespoon low-fat cream cheese (Neufchâtel), softened**
   Chopped fresh chives (optional)
   Freshly ground pepper

Mist nonstick skillet with nonstick cooking spray. Heat the skillet over medium-high heat for 2 minutes. Saute the onion (if using) in hot skillet until tender (2 to 3 minutes). Add smoked salmon to the skillet and stir to mix.

Lightly beat whole egg and egg whites with the cream cheese in a small bowl. Add egg mixture to the salmon mixture in skillet. Stir with a rubber spatula until eggs are set. Sprinkle with the chopped chives, if desired. Season to taste with ground pepper. Serves 1.

Note: If you like, add 1 cooked and crumbled turkey sausage link or slice turkey bacon with the salmon.

South of the Border Tofu Scramble

Nonstick canola oil cooking spray
½ to 1 small serrano chile pepper, seeded and chopped
¼ teaspoon ground cumin
Pinch dried oregano, crushed
1 package (10 ounces) silken tofu, crumbled
¼ cup finely shredded low-fat (2 percent) Monterey Jack cheese
1 tomato, chopped
2 small slices avocado
Chopped cilantro or scallion (optional)

Mist a nonstick skillet with nonstick cooking spray. Heat the skillet over medium-high heat for 2 minutes. Add the chile pepper, cumin, and oregano and saute for 2 minutes or until fragrant. Add tofu and cook until it is hot and has lost some of its moisture. Sprinkle with cheese and turn onto a serving plate. Garnish with tomato and avocado. Top with cilantro or scallion, if desired. Serves 2.

Quick-Fix Egg Scramble

Nonstick canola oil cooking spray
1 **whole egg plus 3 egg whites (or ¾ cup egg substitute or ¾ cup egg purchased egg whites)**
½ **cup chopped fresh, leftover, or frozen and thawed vegetables (such as tomato, broccoli, or any combination of frozen mixed vegetables)**
1 **ounce low-fat (2 percent) cheddar or Monterey Jack cheese or feta cheese, grated (optional if using egg whites)**

Mist a nonstick skillet with nonstick cooking spray. Heat the skillet over medium-high heat for 2 minutes. Lightly beat whole egg and egg whites in a small bowl. Add egg mixture and vegetables to skillet. Stir gently until the eggs are set. Sprinkle with cheese (if using). Serves 1.

Protein Blast Breakfast Scramble

Nonstick canola oil cooking spray
½ **cup sliced fresh mushrooms**
1 **cooked vegetarian sausage patty (such as Morningstar Farms® Veggie Sausage Patty)**
4 **to 6 egg whites (or ¾ cup egg substitute or ¾ cup egg purchased egg whites)**
Bottled hot pepper sauce (optional)

Mist a nonstick skillet with nonstick cooking spray. Heat the skillet over medium-high heat for 2 minutes. Saute mushrooms in hot skillet until they give up some of their moisture (5 minutes). Crumble veggie sausage patty and add to skillet.

Lightly beat egg whites in a small bowl. Add egg whites to skillet. Cook, stirring gently, until mixture is set. Top with a few shakes of bottled hot pepper sauce, if desired. Serves 1.

Western-Style Omelet

Nonstick canola oil cooking spray
¼ **cup chopped green bell pepper**
2 **tablespoons chopped red onion**
1 **whole egg plus 3 egg whites (or ¾ cup egg substitute or purchased egg whites)**
1 **slice low-fat ham, diced**
2 **tablespoons fat-free tomato salsa**
   Bottled hot pepper sauce (optional)

Mist a nonstick skillet with nonstick cooking spray. Heat the skillet over medium-high heat for 2 minutes. Saute bell pepper and onion in hot skillet until tender (2 to 3 minutes). Remove from skillet and set aside.

Lightly beat whole egg and egg whites in a small bowl. Add eggs to the hot skillet. Stir with a rubber spatula, lifting cooked eggs to allow liquid egg to flow underneath. Continue until eggs are almost set and lightly browned on bottom. Place cooked vegetables and the ham on half of the omelet and gently fold over. Tip onto a plate. Top with salsa and, if desired, a few shakes of bottled hot pepper sauce. Serves 1.

Garden Omelet

Nonstick canola oil cooking spray
½ **of a small zucchini, grated or finely chopped**
½ **cup sliced fresh mushrooms**
1 **small tomato, chopped**
½ **teaspoon chopped fresh thyme or ¼ teaspoon dried thyme, crushed**
4 **egg whites (or ¾ cup egg substitute or ¾ cup purchased egg whites)**
1 **whole egg**
Fresh chives, chopped (optional)
Freshly ground pepper

Mist a nonstick skillet with nonstick cooking spray. Heat the skillet over medium-high heat for 2 minutes. Saute zucchini and mushrooms in hot skillet until tender (5 minutes). Add tomato and thyme and heat through for 1 minute. Remove vegetables to a bowl and set aside.

Lightly beat egg whites and whole egg in a small bowl. Add eggs to the hot skillet. Stir with a rubber spatula, lifting cooked eggs to allow liquid egg to flow underneath. Continue until eggs are almost set and lightly browned on bottom. Place cooked vegetables on half of the omelet and gently fold over. Tip onto a serving plate. Sprinkle with chives, if desired. Season to taste with pepper. Serves 1.

The Santa Monica Special

Nonstick canola oil cooking spray
1 **cup packed fresh spinach leaves**
4 **egg whites (or ¾ cup egg substitute or purchased egg whites)**
1 **whole egg**
1 **small tomato, chopped**
½ **of an avocado, chopped**
   Freshly ground pepper

Mist a nonstick skillet with nonstick cooking spray. Heat the skillet over medium-high heat for 2 minutes. Add spinach to hot skillet, cooking and turning with tongs for a few minutes, just until wilted. Remove from skillet and set aside.

Lightly beat egg whites and whole egg in a small bowl. Add eggs to hot skillet. Stir with a rubber spatula, lifting cooked eggs to allow liquid egg to flow underneath. Continue cooking until eggs are almost set and lightly browned on bottom. Place spinach, tomato, and avocado on half of the omelet and gently fold over. Tip onto a serving plate. Season to taste with pepper. Serves 1.

Asparagus Baked Frittata

Nonstick canola oil cooking spray
2 **scallions, chopped**
2 **whole eggs plus 6 egg whites (or 1½ cups egg substitute or purchased egg whites)**
1 **cup low-fat or fat-free ricotta cheese**
Pinch of dried Italian seasoning, crushed
1½ **cups steamed asparagus pieces**

Preheat oven to 425°F.

Mist a small (8-inch) ovenproof nonstick skillet with nonstick cooking spray. Heat skillet over medium-high heat for 2 minutes. Saute the scallions in hot skillet until tender (2 to 3 minutes).

Meanwhile, whisk whole eggs and egg whites, the ricotta cheese, and Italian seasoning in a medium bowl until smooth.

Add the asparagus to the skillet and heat through. Pour egg mixture over the vegetables in skillet. Bake in preheated oven until the eggs are set and the frittata has browned, 25 to 30 minutes. Slice into wedges and serve warm or at room temperature. Serves 2.

Mini Breakfast Frittatas

  Nonstick canola oil cooking spray
4 **ounces lean chicken or turkey sausage, casings removed and meat crumbled**
1 **green or red bell pepper, chopped**
½ **cup sliced fresh mushrooms**
6 **whole eggs (or 2 cups egg substitute)**
3 **tablespoons freshly grated Parmesan cheese**
6 **thin slices tomato**
  Freshly ground pepper

Preheat oven to 350°F. Spray six 1-cup muffin cups with nonstick cooking spray; set aside.

Mist a nonstick skillet with nonstick cooking spray. Heat skillet over medium-high heat for 2 minutes. Add sausage to hot skillet and cook until no longer pink. Drain off fat and place sausage in a bowl.

Saute the bell pepper and mushrooms in the same skillet until tender (2 to 3 minutes). Add to sausage and cool. Stir the eggs and Parmesan cheese into the vegetable mixture. Divide egg mixture evenly among the prepared muffin cups. Place a tomato slice on top of each.

Bake in preheated oven about 20 minutes or until eggs are set. Serve warm or at room temperature. Serves 3 (2 mini frittatas each).

Note: Leftover frittatas can be reheated gently in the microwave; *do not* overcook because the eggs can become rubbery.

Mediterranean Chicken Wrap-Ups

4 **large romaine lettuce leaves**
1 **cooked chicken breast, sliced into strips, or 2 ounces sliced cooked turkey**
¼ **of a cucumber, thinly sliced**
    Grated carrot
¼ **cup feta cheese, crumbled**

Place romaine leaves on a work surface. Divide the chicken strips evenly among the romaine leaves, followed by the cucumber and carrot. Lightly sprinkle feta cheese over each. Tuck in sides and roll up. Serve immediately or wrap individually in plastic wrap and serve later. Serves 1 (4 wrap-ups).

BLT Wrap

1 **low-carb tortilla (such as La Tortilla Factory® or Mission®)**
1 **tablespoon fat-free mayonnaise**
1 **teaspoon Dijon mustard (optional)**
2 **slices roasted turkey breast (3 to 4 ounces)**
2 **large romaine lettuce leaves**
2 **slices tomato**
1 **slice turkey bacon, cooked crisp**
    Freshly ground pepper

Spread tortilla with mayonnaise and, if desired, mustard. Layer turkey, lettuce, tomato, and bacon on half of the wrap. Season to taste with pepper. Roll up tightly, folding in sides as you go. Serve immediately or wrap in plastic wrap and serve later. Serves 1.

Popeye Burgers

1 small onion, finely chopped
2 cloves garlic, finely chopped
2 tablespoons olive oil
1 pound uncooked ground turkey breast
1 teaspoon chopped fresh thyme or ¼ teaspoon dried thyme, crushed
1 teaspoon chopped fresh oregano or ¼ teaspoon dried oregano, crushed
  Dash bottled hot pepper sauce
  Dash ground pepper
1 10-ounce package frozen chopped spinach, thawed and well drained

Cook onion and garlic in hot olive oil in a nonstick skillet over medium heat until tender (5 to 7 minutes). Let cool completely. Place ground turkey in a large bowl; add herbs, bottled hot pepper sauce, and pepper. Add onion mixture to the turkey and mix well. Using your hands, squeeze the spinach to remove excess moisture. Crumble spinach into the turkey mixture; mix until well combined. Shape turkey mixture into 4 patties.

Heat the nonstick skillet over medium-high heat. Cook burgers in the hot skillet for 5 to 7 minutes on each side or until cooked through. Serves 4.

Quick-Fix Sandwich

Spread 2 tablespoons hummus, ricotta cheese, or peanut butter over 1 slice whole grain bread (such as Ezekiel 4:9® or Rudi's Organic Bakery®). Top with veggies (lettuce, chopped cucumber, chopped tomato, chopped bell pepper). Season to taste with freshly ground pepper. Serves 1.

Niçoise Roll-Ups

1   hard-cooked egg white, chopped
    Niçoise Salad Dressing (recipe follows)
4   Boston lettuce leaves
4   to 6 ounces water-pack tuna (in can or pouch)
½   cup blanched green beans (or any leftover cooked green vegetable)
6   cherry tomatoes

Mix egg white with Niçoise Salad Dressing and spread over lettuce leaves.
Drain tuna and flake with a fork. Divide tuna and green beans among the
lettuce leaves. Roll up tightly. Wrap roll-ups individually in plastic wrap to
keep them together. Serve the cherry tomatoes on the side. Serves 1.

Niçoise Salad Dressing

1   tablespoon Dijon mustard
3   tablespoons fresh lemon juice
    Pinch dried thyme, crushed
2   tablespoons fat-free mayonnaise
1   tablespoon capers

Whisk together Dijon mustard, lemon juice, and thyme in a small bowl. Whisk
in the mayonnaise and the capers. Let rest to blend flavors.
*Or try Follow Your Heart® low-fat Ranch dressing (25 calories per
2 tablespoons).*

Hummus in Pita

1 whole wheat pita (such as Ezekiel 4:9®), cut crosswise in half
¼ cup hummus
4 cucumber slices
2 tomato slices
2 radishes, thinly sliced (optional)

Carefully open pita bread to make pockets. Spread hummus inside and arrange vegetables in the pockets. Serves 1.

Grilled Chicken Salad

2 grilled skinless, boneless chicken breast halves
8 cups torn salad greens
½ of a cucumber, thinly sliced
1 large tomato, cut into wedges
½ of a green or red bell pepper, cut into matchsticks
2 scallions, sliced
  Salad Dressing (choose one from the dressings listed on pages 199 to 201)
½ of an avocado, peeled and diced
2 hard-cooked egg whites, chopped (optional)

Cut chicken into bite-size pieces; set aside. Mix the salad greens, cucumber, tomato, bell pepper, and scallions in a large bowl. Toss with the dressing and divide between 2 bowls. Sprinkle the avocado and, if desired, egg whites over the salad. Arrange chicken pieces on each salad. Serves 2.

LUNCH

Curried Chicken Salad in Papaya

½ cup plain fat-free yogurt
½ teaspoon mild curry powder (or more to taste)
8 ounces cooked chicken or turkey breast or cooked small shrimp
½ of an apple, chopped
1 ripe papaya, halved and seeded (or ½ of a cantaloupe)
2 teaspoons chopped fresh cilantro
   Lime wedges

Mix yogurt with curry powder until well blended. Taste and, if desired, add more curry. Fold chicken and apple into yogurt mixture. Scoop chicken mixture into each papaya half and garnish with chopped cilantro. Serve lime wedges on the side. Serves 2.

Quick-Fix Salad

Place 3 to 4 cups of any torn salad greens in a bowl. Add 4 to 5 ounces cooked meat (chicken, turkey, canned tuna). Dress with 2 tablespoons low-fat dressing. Season to taste with freshly ground pepper. Serves 1.

Farmer's Market Chopped Salad

- **4 cups** chopped firm salad greens, such as romaine lettuce (preferably organic)
- **½ cup** chopped jicama
- **½ cup** chopped red bell pepper
- **½ cup** chopped, seeded cucumber
- **1 carrot,** chopped
- **2 scallions,** chopped
- **4 dried apricots,** snipped with scissors into small pieces
  Creamy Buttermilk Dressing (page 201) or other salad dressing (see pages 199 to 201)
- **2 cooked** skinless, boneless chicken breast halves, cut into small cubes, 1 cup cubed cooked turkey, or 2 to 4 ounces sliced turkey breast from the deli, chopped
- **¼ cup** feta cheese, crumbled (optional)

Mix greens, jicama, bell pepper, cucumber, carrot, scallions, and apricots in a large bowl. Toss with dressing. Fold in chicken. Sprinkle with feta cheese, if desired. Serves 2.

Chinese Chicken Salad

3 cups torn romaine lettuce
2 cups finely shredded napa cabbage
½ cup shredded carrot
½ cup bean sprouts
2 scallions, sliced
¼ cup chopped cilantro
   Chinese Chicken Salad Dressing (page 201)
2 4-ounce skinless, boneless chicken breast halves, cooked and thinly sliced
2 tablespoons slivered almonds (optional)
   Lime wedges (optional)

Toss lettuce, cabbage, carrot, bean sprouts, scallions, and cilantro in a large
bowl. Add dressing and toss again to blend. Divide between 2 plates. Top with
sliced chicken and, if desired, sprinkle with almonds. Serve lime wedges on
the side, if desired. Serves 2.

Edamame and Spinach Salad

1 **9-ounce package prewashed baby spinach leaves**
1 **cup cooked shelled edamame (green soybeans)***
1 **cup shredded cooked chicken**
½ **cup bean sprouts**
¼ **cup grated carrot**
2 **tablespoons rice vinegar**
1 **tablespoon low-sodium soy sauce**
1 **teaspoon dark sesame oil**
   Toasted sesame seeds (optional)

Toss spinach with edamame in a large salad bowl. Arrange chicken, bean sprouts, and carrot attractively on top. For dressing, whisk together rice vinegar, soy sauce, and sesame oil in a small bowl. Drizzle dressing over salad. Sprinkle with sesame seeds, if desired. Serves 2.

*Note: Shelled edamame are now available in the frozen food section of many markets.

Blue Plate Turkey Burger Salad

½ of a red bell pepper, chopped
1 shallot, chopped
2 tablespoons canola oil, divided
1 pound uncooked ground turkey (not all breast meat)
½ teaspoon salt-free seasoning (such as Mrs. Dash®)
   Freshly ground pepper
6 to 8 cups roughly torn romaine lettuce leaves
1 large tomato, sliced
½ of an avocado, sliced

Cook bell pepper and shallot in 1 tablespoon hot oil in a skillet over medium-high heat until tender (3 to 5 minutes). Transfer to a large bowl and let cool. Add turkey and salt-free seasoning to the bell pepper mixture and mix gently; season to taste with pepper. Form mixture into 2 patties.

Heat the remaining 1 tablespoon oil in the same skillet. Add the patties to the hot skillet and cook, turning once, for a total of 9 minutes or until done. Divide lettuce between 2 plates. Place a burger on each plate. Arrange tomato and avocado slices around the burgers. Serves 2.

Tuscan Bean and Tuna Salad

7   **ounces water-pack tuna (in a can or pouch), drained**
1   **cup cooked green beans**
½   **cup canned cannellini beans, rinsed and drained (or shelled edamame)**
2   **tablespoons extra virgin olive oil**
2   **tablespoons fresh lemon juice**
6   **cups torn salad greens**
2   **tablespoons chopped parsley**
2   **scallions, chopped (optional)**

Place tuna in a large bowl; flake with a fork. Add green beans and cannellini beans to tuna. Drizzle with olive oil and lemon juice and toss gently to coat. Arrange salad greens on 2 plates. Divide tuna mixture and place on top of salad greens. Garnish with a sprinkling of parsley and, if desired, scallions. Serves 2.

Salmon Salad with Miso Dressing

6   **cups torn salad greens**
1   **cup assorted vegetables (such as chopped cucumber, shredded carrots, bean sprouts)**
1   **7-ounce pouch water-pack salmon or leftover cooked salmon fillet**
6   **tablespoons Miso Dressing (page 200)**
   Toasted sesame seeds (optional)

Arrange salad greens and vegetables on 2 large plates. Flake salmon over the top. Drizzle 3 tablespoons of dressing over each salad. Sprinkle with sesame seeds, if desired. Serves 2.

Thai Beef Salad

2 tablespoons low-sodium soy sauce
1 pound flank steak
  Freshly ground pepper
6 to 8 cups torn salad greens
½ of a hothouse cucumber, sliced thin
1 red bell pepper, cut into strips
4 scallions, sliced
1 cup snipped fresh herb mixture containing basil, mint, and cilantro
  Thai Salad Dressing (page 199)
2 tablespoons chopped pine nuts (optional)

For the meat, preheat a grill pan or broiler. Drizzle the soy sauce on both sides of the flank steak and sprinkle with ground pepper. Grill or broil steak to desired doneness. Let steak rest while you prepare the salad.

For the salad, place salad greens, cucumber, bell pepper, scallions, and herb mixture in a large bowl. Slice the steak across the grain into thin strips. Mound the steak on top of the salad. Drizzle with the dressing. Sprinkle with pine nuts, if desired. Serves 4.

Quick-Fix Lunch Plate

Place 4 to 5 ounces of cooked meat (chicken, turkey, canned tuna) on a plate. Add 1 or 2 steamed vegetables (broccoli, spinach, asparagus, green beans). Season to taste with freshly ground pepper. Serves 1.

Vinaigrette Dressing

2   tablespoons balsamic vinegar
1   teaspoon Dijon mustard
1   teaspoon finely chopped shallot or chives (optional)
2   tablespoons olive oil
    Freshly ground pepper to taste

Whisk the vinegar and mustard in a bowl. Add shallot, if desired. Slowly whisk in the olive oil until well incorporated. Season to taste with pepper. Let stand for a few minutes to blend flavors. Serves 2.
Or try Annie's Naturals® low-fat Raspberry Vinaigrette (35 calories per 2 tablespoons).

LUNCH

Thai Salad Dressing

¼   cup fish sauce (Thai *nam pla*) or low-sodium soy sauce
¼   cup fresh lime juice
1   serrano chile pepper, minced
4   teaspoons sugar or honey

Mix all ingredients in a small bowl; let rest to blend flavors. Serves 4.
Or try Annie's Naturals® Gingerly Vinaigrette (40 calories per 2 tablespoons).

Miso Dressing

4½ tablespoons yellow miso (soybean paste)
4½ tablespoons honey
  3 tablespoons rice vinegar
  3 tablespoons mustard (Dijon or other spicy style)

Whisk together all ingredients in a small bowl until smooth. Store in refrigerator. Serves 6.
Or try Annie's Naturals® low-fat Honey Mustard Vinaigrette (45 calories per 2 tablespoons).

Caesar Salad Dressing

  1 tablespoon low-fat mayonnaise
  1 teaspoon freshly grated Parmesan cheese
  1 teaspoon fresh lemon juice
  ½ teaspoon capers, drained (optional)
  ½ teaspoon Dijon mustard
    Dash Worcestershire sauce
    Freshly ground pepper

Mix all ingredients in a bowl. Serves 1.
Or try Follow Your Heart® Caesar Dressing (80 calories per 2 tablespoons).

Chinese Chicken Salad Dressing

1 **quarter-size piece peeled fresh ginger**
1 **small shallot, peeled and cut into quarters**
2 **tablespoons low-sodium soy sauce**
1 **tablespoon canola oil**
1 **tablespoon rice wine vinegar**
1 **heaping teaspoon Dijon mustard**
1 **teaspoon honey**
1 **teaspoon toasted sesame oil**
  A few drops hot chili oil (optional)

Using a mini food processor, finely mince ginger and shallot. Add remaining ingredients and process until blended. (Or finely chop ginger and shallot; whisk in the remaining ingredients.) Serves 2.
Or try Annie's Naturals® low-fat Gingerly Vinaigrette (40 calories per 2 tablespoons).

Creamy Buttermilk Dressing

4 **tablespoons fat-free buttermilk**
⅓ **cup part-skim ricotta cheese**
1 **teaspoon Dijon mustard**
¼ **teaspoon minced garlic (½ of a small clove)**
1 **tablespoon fresh lemon juice**
1 **tablespoon chopped chives**
  Freshly ground pepper

Whisk buttermilk, ricotta cheese, mustard, garlic, lemon juice, and chives in a bowl until well combined. Season to taste with pepper. Serves 4.
Or try Follow Your Heart® low-fat Ranch Dressing (25 calories per 2 tablespoons).

Chili-Rubbed Chicken Breasts with Mango Salsa

4 skinless, boneless chicken breast halves
½ cup fresh orange juice
2 tablespoons fresh lime juice
1 small clove garlic, chopped
   Nonstick canola oil cooking spray
1 tablespoon mild chili powder
   Mango Salsa (recipe, page 217)

Place chicken breast halves between sheets of plastic wrap. Flatten chicken slightly with the palm of your hand or a heavy skillet.* Mix orange juice, lime juice, and garlic in a glass dish. Add chicken; cover and marinate in the refrigerator for 2 hours.

Remove chicken from marinade and pat dry. Discard marinade. Lightly spray chicken on both sides with nonstick cooking spray. Sprinkle chili powder on both sides of chicken.

Preheat grill pan or nonstick skillet over medium-high heat. When pan is hot, add chicken and sear on one side for 5 minutes. Turn chicken over and cook for 5 minutes more or until cooked through. Serve chicken with the Mango Salsa. Serves 4.

*Note: Flattening the chicken breasts between sheets of plastic wrap with the palm of your hand or a heavy skillet helps them to cook more evenly. If you prefer, substitute 1 pound turkey breast cutlets for the chicken.

DINNER

Tuscan Chicken

For the marinade:
- **2 tablespoons olive oil**
- **1 tablespoon chopped fresh rosemary**
- **1 tablespoon chopped fresh sage leaves**
- **Zest of 1 lemon**
- **Juice of 1 lemon**
- **2 cloves garlic, minced**
- **Freshly ground pepper**

For the chicken:
- **4 skinless, boneless chicken breast halves**
- **4 roma tomatoes, seeded and chopped**
- **1 tablespoon capers, drained**
- **1 tablespoon chopped kalamata olives**
- **Chopped fresh parsley**

For the marinade, mix together olive oil, rosemary, sage, lemon zest, lemon juice, and garlic in a large nonreactive bowl. Add freshly ground pepper to taste. Set aside.

Place chicken breast halves between sheets of plastic wrap. Flatten chicken slightly with the palm of your hand or a heavy skillet (see Note, page 202). Place chicken in a glass dish; add marinade. Cover and marinate in the refrigerator for 2 to 4 hours.

Remove chicken from marinade and pat dry. Discard marinade. Heat a nonstick skillet over medium-high heat. Add chicken and cook for 5 minutes on one side. Turn and cook for 5 minutes more or until cooked through. Remove chicken to a warm plate. Add chopped tomatoes, capers, and olives to skillet and cook a few minutes or until tomatoes start to break down. Top chicken with hot tomato mixture and sprinkle with parsley. Serves 4.

DINNER

Chicken Skewers

¼ cup red wine vinegar
¼ cup olive oil
1 tablespoon low-sodium soy sauce
½ teaspoon dried oregano
    Pinch red pepper flakes
1 clove garlic, minced
4 skinless, boneless chicken breast halves, cut into 1-inch chunks
1 large green or red bell pepper, cut into 1-inch chunks
    Bamboo skewers soaked in water for 30 minutes

For marinade, mix vinegar, olive oil, soy sauce, oregano, red pepper flakes, and garlic in a nonreactive dish. Add chicken pieces to the marinade. Cover and marinate in the refrigerator for 1 hour.

Remove chicken from the marinade. Discard marinade. Thread chicken and bell pepper alternately on skewers, taking care not to pack the pieces too closely together.

Preheat grill to medium-high heat or broiler to high heat. Grill or broil the skewers for 5 minutes on each side or until chicken is cooked through. Serves 4.

Spicy Oven-Fried Chicken

3 tablespoons bottled hot pepper sauce
1 tablespoon Worcestershire sauce
1 teaspoon salt (optional)
1 teaspoon freshly ground pepper
8 chicken pieces (breast halves, thighs, and/or drumsticks)
2 cups unseasoned bread crumbs
1 to 2 tablespoons vegetable oil (such as canola, safflower, or sunflower)

Whisk together bottled hot pepper sauce, Worcestershire sauce, salt (if desired), and pepper in a rectangular baking dish. Add the chicken, turning to coat. Cover and marinate in the refrigerator for 2 to 24 hours.

Preheat the oven to 425°F. Remove the chicken from the marinade and add the bread crumbs to the marinade. Mix well; pat the crumb mixture onto the chicken.

Spread the oil over the bottom of a shallow 3-quart rectangular baking dish. Arrange the chicken in the dish. Bake for 15 to 20 minutes in the preheated oven. Turn the chicken over; reduce the heat to 325° and bake for 15 to 20 minutes more, or until the juices run clear when chicken is pierced with a fork. Serves 8.

DINNER

Turkey Meatballs Marinara

1   pound uncooked ground turkey (not too lean)
1   egg, lightly beaten
3   tablespoons purchased basil pesto
3   to 4 tablespoons dry bread crumbs
**   Freshly ground pepper**
1   28-ounce jar low-fat tomato pasta sauce
3   tablespoons freshly grated Parmesan cheese (optional)

Mix turkey, egg, and pesto in a large bowl. Add 3 tablespoons bread crumbs and mix well. If mixture seems too moist, add the remaining tablespoon of bread crumbs. Add pepper to taste.

Pour pasta sauce into a 10-inch skillet with a lid and bring to a simmer over medium heat. Moisten hands with cold water and roll turkey mixture into golf ball-size meatballs and place gently in hot pasta sauce (you should have 12 to 14 meatballs). Cover and simmer for 30 minutes or until cooked through, shaking the pan halfway through cooking to roll over the meatballs. Transfer meatballs and sauce to a serving plate. Sprinkle with Parmesan cheese, if desired. Serves 2 to 3.

New Orleans-Style Halibut

Nonstick canola oil cooking spray
4 **halibut fillets (4 to 6 ounces each)**
1 **tablespoon Dijon mustard**
2 **teaspoons canola oil**
½ **teaspoon Cajun-style seasoning**
 Chopped scallions (optional)
 Lemon wedges

Preheat oven to 425°F. Mist a foil-lined baking sheet with nonstick cooking spray. Place fish on baking sheet. Mix mustard, canola oil, and Cajun seasoning in a small bowl. Spread mustard mixture evenly over fish. Bake in preheated oven for 15 minutes or until fish is cooked through. Sprinkle with scallions, if desired. Serve with lemon wedges. Serves 4.

Steamed Fish with Chinese Herbs

2 **tablespoons low-sodium soy sauce**
1 **tablespoon dry sherry or white wine**
1 **teaspoon toasted sesame oil**
12 **ounces fish fillets (such as red snapper or rock cod)**
2 **tablespoons grated fresh ginger**
 Freshly ground pepper
3 **scallions, slivered**
¼ **cup chopped fresh cilantro (optional)**

Mix soy sauce, sherry, and sesame oil in small bowl. Rub fish with the soy sauce mixture and place in a glass pie plate. Sprinkle ginger evenly over the fish. Sprinkle fish with pepper to taste. Bring water to boiling in a steamer (either a Chinese bamboo steamer or a large pot with a steamer insert that will hold the plate with the fish). Place fish above the steam; cover and cook for 6 to 8 minutes or until fish is cooked through. Sprinkle with the scallions and, if desired, cilantro. Serves 2.

DINNER

Asian Glazed Salmon

3 tablespoons white or yellow miso (soybean paste)
2 tablespoons minced fresh ginger
2 tablespoons brown sugar
2 tablespoons low-sodium soy sauce
2 tablespoons water
   Nonstick canola oil cooking spray
4 salmon fillets (4 to 6 ounces each)
   Chopped scallions

Preheat broiler. Stir together miso, ginger, brown sugar, soy sauce, and water in a small bowl, mixing until well combined. Line a baking sheet with foil and mist with nonstick cooking spray. Arrange fish on baking sheet, skin sides down. Coat each piece with the miso mixture. Broil fish 6 inches from heat for 10 minutes or until fish is cooked through. Sprinkle with scallions. Serves 4.

Broiled Salmon Dijonnaise

2 tablespoons whole grain mustard
2 tablespoons light mayonnaise
½ teaspoon chopped fresh thyme
½ teaspoon chopped fresh rosemary
1 clove garlic, minced
4 salmon fillets (4 to 6 ounces each)
   Freshly ground pepper
   Lemon wedges

Preheat broiler. Mix mustard, mayonnaise, thyme, rosemary, and garlic in a small bowl. Line a baking sheet with foil. Place salmon fillets, skin sides down, on foil. Coat the top of each fillet with the mustard mixture. Broil the fish 6 inches from heat for 5 to 7 minutes or until the tops are browned. Check for doneness; if the fish needs to cook a little longer, turn off broiler and let stand in hot oven for a few more minutes until cooked through. Season to taste with pepper. Serve with lemon wedges. Serves 4.

DINNER

Tilapia Saute with Greens

2 tablespoons olive oil, divided
2 cloves garlic, finely chopped
1 large bunch Swiss chard, ribs and stems removed, chopped coarsely
1 large shallot, thinly sliced
8 to 12 ounces tilapia fillets (or other thin white fish fillets)
2 tablespoons fresh lemon juice
Freshly ground pepper

Heat 1 tablespoon of the olive oil in a very large nonstick skillet. Add garlic and saute for less than a minute (do not let it brown). Start adding the Swiss chard to the skillet in large handfuls, stirring just until chard begins to wilt. Keep adding the chard until all is in the pan, cooking and turning just until tender. Remove chard to a plate and keep warm.

Heat the remaining 1 tablespoon olive oil in the same skillet. Add the shallot and saute until tender. Add fish to skillet and cook over medium-high heat until browned on each side and cooked through, 6 minutes total. Sprinkle with lemon juice; season to taste with pepper. Serves 2.

Fish in a Packet

4 cups fresh spinach (packaged spinach is a timesaver)
4 fish fillets such as cod, sea bass, or halibut (4 to 6 ounces each)
½ cup white wine or chicken broth
1½ tablespoons olive oil
4 lemon slices
1 tablespoon minced garlic
Freshly ground pepper

Preheat the oven to 375°F. Cut four 12-inch squares of foil. Divide spinach among foil squares. Top with a piece of fish. Distribute the wine, olive oil, lemon, and garlic evenly over the fish. Gather up the sides of each foil square to form a packet and fold the edges over tightly to seal. Place the packets on a baking sheet. Bake in preheated oven for 15 to 20 minutes, depending on the thickness of the fish. Transfer packets to plates; open carefully. Season to taste with pepper. Serves 4.

Vietnamese-Style Grilled Flank Steak With Portobello Mushrooms

For the marinade:

- **4 tablespoons low-sodium soy sauce**
- **1 tablespoon grated fresh ginger**
- **1 tablespoon honey**
- **1 tablespoon toasted sesame oil**
- **1 teaspoon minced garlic**

For the meat:

- **1 pound flank steak**
- **2 large portobello mushrooms, stems removed, gills scraped clean**
- **Canola oil for brushing on grill**
- **¼ cup chopped scallions**
- **¼ cup chopped fresh mint**
- **¼ cup chopped fresh cilantro**
- **Lime wedges**

For the marinade, mix together soy sauce, ginger, honey, sesame oil, and garlic in a small bowl.

Place steak and mushrooms in a rectangular baking dish. Drizzle marinade over steak and mushrooms. Cover and marinate in the refrigerator for 1 hour. Prepare grill (or use an indoor grill pan). Remove steak and mushrooms from marinade. Discard marinade.

Brush grill rack or grill pan lightly with oil and grill steak for 4 minutes on each side or until desired doneness. Remove steak from grill or pan and let rest, covered with foil, while you grill the mushrooms for 3 minutes on each side. Slice the steak thinly across the grain and slice the mushrooms into thick pieces. Arrange on plates and sprinkle with scallions, mint, and cilantro. Serve lime wedges on the side. Serves 4.

Curry Burgers

1 **pound lean ground beef or ground uncooked turkey**
¼ **cup finely chopped onion**
¼ **cup finely chopped cilantro**
1 **fresh serrano chile pepper, seeded and finely chopped (optional)**
1 **tablespoon ground cumin**
1 **tablespoon ground ginger**
1 **tablespoon curry powder**
¼ **teaspoon ground cinnamon**
  Nonstick canola oil cooking spray
  Mango Salsa (recipe, page 217)

Combine beef, onion, cilantro, chile pepper (if desired), cumin, ginger, curry powder, and cinnamon in a large bowl; mix well. Shape beef mixture into 4 patties.

Mist a nonstick skillet with nonstick cooking spray. Heat the skillet over medium-high heat for 2 minutes. Cook patties in hot skillet for 4 to 5 minutes on each side or until cooked through. Top each burger with Mango Salsa. Serves 4.

DINNER

Broccoli-Tofu Stir-Fry

¼ cup tamari or light soy sauce
3 tablespoons sesame seeds, divided
2 tablespoons brown rice vinegar
1 tablespoon honey
1 tablespoon toasted sesame oil
1 pound firm tofu
1 tablespoon extra virgin olive oil or toasted sesame oil
4 tablespoons minced fresh ginger
4 large garlic cloves, minced
½ of a medium white onion, sliced lengthwise into crescents
2 carrots, cut diagonally into ½-inch pieces
1 cup sliced mushrooms
1½ cups broccoli florets
2 cups chopped Chinese greens, such as bok choy or napa cabbage
½ of a small red or yellow bell pepper, cut into strips
½ cup chopped red cabbage
   Hot cooked brown rice

For the sauce, combine the tamari, 2 tablespoons of the sesame seeds, rice vinegar, honey, and sesame oil in a small bowl. Set sauce aside.

Cut tofu into bite-size pieces; set aside. Heat the olive oil in large skillet or wok over medium-high heat. Add the ginger and garlic and cook for 2 to 3 minutes. Add the onion, carrots, and tofu and cook for 2 minutes.

Reduce the heat to medium. Add the mushrooms and cook for 3 minutes or until the onion is transparent. Add the broccoli and cook for 2 to 3 minutes. Add the greens, bell pepper, and red cabbage and cook for 2 minutes more.

Add the sauce to the vegetable mixture in the skillet and cook for 4 to 5 minutes over low heat. Serve stir-fry with brown rice. Sprinkle with the remaining 1 tablespoon sesame seeds. Serves 4.

Master Recipe for Stir-Fry

Use these proportions to create your own signature stir-fry dishes.

4 **tablespoons canola oil, divided**
1 **pound vegetables, cut into 1-inch pieces (use a mixture, such as broccoli, mushrooms, and bell peppers)**
1 **pound meat/poultry/seafood, cut into 1-inch pieces**
1 **tablespoon minced fresh ginger**
1 **to 2 cloves garlic, minced**
Desired stir-fry sauce

Heat wok or large skillet over high heat. Add 2 tablespoons of the oil and heat until almost smoking. Add the vegetables and stir-fry 3 to 5 minutes. Remove from wok. Add 1 to 2 tablespoons more oil to the wok as needed; add meat and cook for 2 to 3 minutes. Add the ginger and garlic; cook and stir until the meat is almost done. Return veggies to wok and cook 1 minute to heat through. Stir in your choice of stir-fry sauce. Serves 4.

Black Bean Stir-Fry Sauce: Combine 1½ tablespoons cornstarch and 1 tablespoon water in a small saucepan; stir until smooth. Stir in ¼ cup black bean sauce, ¾ cup low-fat/low-sodium chicken broth, 1 tablespoon minced fresh ginger, and ¼ cup chopped scallions. Cook and stir until thickened (3 to 4 minutes).

Spicy Garlic Stir-Fry Sauce: Combine 1 tablespoon water and 1 teaspoon cornstarch in a small saucepan. Stir in ½ cup low-fat/low-sodium chicken broth, 1½ tablespoons low-sodium soy sauce, 1½ teaspoons chili garlic sauce, 1 tablespoon ketchup, and 1 tablespoon dry sherry or red wine. Cook and stir until thickened (3 to 4 minutes).

Thai Stir-Fry Sauce: Stir together 1 tablespoon water and 1 teaspoon cornstarch in a small saucepan. Stir in ½ cup low-fat/low-sodium chicken broth; 1 clove garlic, minced; 3 tablespoons Thai fish sauce or low-sodium fish sauce; 1 tablespoon honey; ½ to 1 serrano chile pepper, finely chopped; and 1 tablespoon lime juice. Cook and stir until thickened.

DINNER

Grilled Chicken Breasts

4 skinless, boneless chicken breast halves or turkey cutlets (1 pound total)
2 tablespoons olive oil or canola oil
1 tablespoon seasoning (mild chili powder, curry powder, Italian herb mix, jerk seasoning, Cajun seasoning, or low-sodium soy sauce)

Flatten chicken slightly with the palm of your hand or a heavy skillet (see Note, page 202). Rub chicken breast halves with the oil and sprinkle on both sides with the seasoning of your choice. Let rest while you heat a grill pan, a barbecue grill, or a heavy nonstick skillet to medium-high. Cook chicken on each side for 4 to 5 minutes or until golden brown and cooked through. Serve with any of the salsas on pages 215 to 217. Serves 4.

DINNER

Salsa Toppers for Chicken

Pico de Gallo

2 large ripe tomatoes, chopped
4 tablespoons chopped fresh cilantro
2 scallions, chopped
2 tablespoons fresh lime juice
  Freshly ground black pepper

Combine tomatoes, cilantro, scallions, and lime juice in a bowl. Season to taste with pepper. Let stand to blend flavors.

Tomato-Basil Salsa Fresca

2 large ripe tomatoes, chopped
4 tablespoons chopped fresh basil
1 tablespoon balsamic vinegar
1 tablespoon capers, drained (optional)
  Freshly ground pepper

Combine tomatoes, basil, vinegar, and, if desired, capers in a bowl. Season to taste with pepper. Let stand to blend flavors.

Cucumber Salsa

2 tablespoons seasoned rice vinegar
  Pinch red pepper flakes
1 hothouse cucumber, seeded and thinly sliced
½ of a red bell pepper, chopped

Combine rice vinegar, red pepper flakes, cucumber, and bell pepper in a bowl. Let stand to blend flavors.

DINNER

Pineapple Salsa

2 **cups chopped fresh pineapple**
½ **of a jalapeño chile pepper, seeded and chopped**
½ **of a red onion, chopped**
2 **tablespoons fresh lime juice**

Combine pineapple, chile pepper, onion, and lime juice in a bowl. Let stand to blend flavors.

Melon Salsa

2 **cups diced melon (cantaloupe, honeydew, etc.)**
3 **tablespoons chopped fresh mint**
2 **tablespoons fresh lime juice**
½ **teaspoon freshly grated ginger**
½ **of a jalapeño pepper, finely chopped (optional)**

Combine melon, mint, lime juice, ginger, and, if desired, jalapeño pepper in a bowl. Let stand to blend flavors.

Avocado-Jicama Salsa

1 **avocado, peeled and diced**
1 **cup diced jicama**
2 **tablespoons fresh lime juice**
3 **tablespoons chopped cilantro**

Combine avocado, jicama, lime juice, and cilantro in a bowl. Let stand to blend flavors.

Papaya Salsa

1 ripe papaya, peeled, seeded, and diced
½ of a red bell pepper, diced
1 teaspoon grated lime zest
2 tablespoons fresh lime juice
2 tablespoons chopped scallion or chives

Combine papaya, bell pepper, lime zest, lime juice, and scallion in a bowl. Let stand to blend flavors.

Raita

1 hothouse cucumber, peeled, seeded, and diced
1 cup fat-free plain yogurt (preferably Greek style)
1 teaspoon kosher salt
1 clove garlic, minced
¼ teaspoon ground cumin
   Cayenne pepper (optional)

Sprinkle cucumber with salt in a strainer and let rest for 30 minutes. Meanwhile, combine yogurt, salt, garlic, and cumin in a bowl. Rinse cucumber under running water and squeeze dry in a paper towel. Add cucumber to yogurt mixture. Stir to blend. Season to taste with cayenne pepper, if desired.

Mango Salsa

1 large ripe mango, peeled, seeded, and diced
2 tablespoons fresh lime juice
1 small red bell pepper, cut into small dice
2 scallions, chopped
2 tablespoons chopped cilantro
   Cayenne pepper

Combine mango, lime juice, bell pepper, scallions, and cilantro in a bowl. Season to taste with cayenne pepper. Let stand to blend flavors.

DINNER

Acorn Squash with Rosemary

2   acorn squash, cut into 4 wedges each
4   tablespoons balsamic vinegar
2   tablespoons olive oil
4   sprigs fresh rosemary
    Freshly ground pepper

Preheat oven to 425°F. Toss squash wedges with vinegar, oil, and rosemary. Sprinkle with pepper to taste. Place on a baking sheet. Roast in preheated oven for 30 to 40 minutes, turning pieces over halfway through roasting. Serves 4.

Roasted Asparagus with Lemon

1   pound asparagus spears
1   tablespoon olive oil
    Freshly ground pepper
1   lemon, cut into 4 wedges
1   tablespoon freshly grated Parmesan cheese (optional)

Preheat oven to 425°F. Toss asparagus with olive oil and pepper to taste. Place in a single layer on a baking sheet. Roast in preheated oven for 15 to 20 minutes, shaking pan halfway through to turn asparagus over. Squeeze lemon wedges over asparagus. Sprinkle with Parmesan cheese, if desired. Serves 4.

SIDES

Roasted Mushrooms with Garlic

1 pound cremini mushrooms, thickly sliced
2 tablespoons olive oil
2 tablespoons chopped parsley
1 large clove garlic, minced
   Pinch red pepper flakes (optional)

Preheat oven to 425°F. Toss mushroom slices with olive oil and arrange on a baking sheet. Roast in preheated oven for 15 to 20 minutes, stirring once halfway through roasting. Transfer mushrooms to a bowl and toss with the parsley and garlic. Sprinkle with red pepper flakes, if desired. Serves 4.

Roasted Green Beans with Almonds

1 pound green beans, ends trimmed
1 large shallot, thinly sliced
1 tablespoon olive oil
¼ cup slivered almonds

SIDES

Preheat oven to 425°F. Toss green beans and shallot with olive oil. Arrange beans and shallot on a baking sheet. Roast in preheated oven for 10 to 15 minutes. During the last 5 minutes of roasting, add the slivered almonds; toss to mix. Continue roasting until beans are tender and almonds are golden. Serves 4.

Cauliflower Mashed Potatoes

1   **cup mashed steamed cauliflower**
2   **tablespoons Smart Balance® Buttery Spread**
½   **cup shredded low-fat mozzarella cheese**
    Dash salt and ground pepper

Preheat oven to 400°F. Stir together mashed cauliflower, buttery spread, cheese, salt, and pepper. Spoon into a small baking dish. Bake in preheated oven about 15 minutes or until heated through. Serves 2.

Zucchini Chips

1   **cup sliced zucchini**
1   **tablespoon olive oil**
    Garlic salt
    Grated Parmesan cheese

Preheat oven to 400°F. Spread zucchini on baking sheet. Drizzle with olive oil. Sprinkle with garlic salt and Parmesan cheese. Bake in preheated oven for 15 to 20 minutes or until crisp-tender. Serves 2.

Green Beans, Chinese-Style

1   **cup trimmed green beans**
2   **tablespoons plum sauce**
1   **tablespoon canola oil**

Preheat grill. Toss green beans with plum sauce and oil in a bowl. Grill, covered, over low heat about 10 minutes or until tender. Serves 2.

SIDES

Green Beans, French-Style

1 **cup green beans, steamed just until crisp-tender**
 Nonstick canola oil cooking spray
 Paprika
 Garlic salt

Preheat oven to 400°F. Place green beans on a baking sheet. Mist green beans with nonstick cooking spray. Sprinkle with paprika and garlic salt. Bake about 10 minutes or until beans are lightly browned. Serves 2.

Grilled Asparagus with Dried Tomatoes

 Nonstick cooking spray
8 **asparagus spears**
¼ **cup snipped dried tomatoes**

Mist grill rack with nonstick cooking spray. Preheat grill. Grill asparagus over medium heat for 8 to minutes or until crisp-tender. Sprinkle with tomatoes. Serves 2.

SIDES

Prosciutto-Wrapped Asparagus

8 **asparagus spears, steamed**
3 **ounces prosciutto**

Preheat oven to 400°F. Wrap 2 asparagus spears in one-fourth of the prosciutto. Repeat with remaining asparagus and prosciutto. Arrange in shallow baking pan and bake in preheated oven for 10 to 15 minutes or until asparagus is lightly browned. Serves 2.

Turkey Bacon-Wrapped Asparagus

3 to 6 slices turkey bacon
8 asparagus spears, steamed

Preheat oven to 400°F. Wrap turkey bacon around 2 asparagus spears; place in shallow baking pan. Repeat to make 4 asparagus bundles. Bake in preheated oven for 10 to 15 minutes. Serves 2.

Broccoli & Spinach Fix-Ups

Broccoli

• Toss 1 cup cooked broccoli with dried tomatoes, grated Parmesan cheese, and 1 teaspoon olive oil.

• Toss 1 cup stir-fried broccoli with low-sodium soy sauce and grated Parmesan cheese.

• Toss 1 cup cooked broccoli with 1 tablespoon Smart Balance® Buttery Spread, 1 minced garlic clove, and ¼ cup dry white wine.

• Toss 1 cup cooked broccoli with ½ cup tomato sauce and ¼ cup shredded mozzarella cheese. Heat to melt cheese.

Spinach

• Toss 1 cup fresh spinach with 1 tablespoon olive oil, ¼ cup crumbled feta cheese, and 1 minced garlic clove.

• Combine 1 cup fresh spinach, ½ cup low-fat milk, ¼ cup fat-free cottage or ricotta cheese, salt, and ground pepper in a small casserole. Bake in preheated 350°F oven for 15 minutes or until it's nice and crunchy on top.

• Top 1 cup fresh spinach with ¼ cup pine nuts and ¼ cup ricotta cheese.

Note: When you cook your vegetables, you increase the level of vitamin C. For example, 1 cup of raw broccoli contains 20 mg of vitamin C. If you microwave it for 1½ minutes, you increase the vitamin C level to 43 mg. Just be sure not to overcook!

Brown Rice

$3\frac{1}{2}$ **cups low-fat chicken or vegetable broth or water**
$\frac{1}{2}$ **teaspoon salt (optional)**
2 **cups uncooked brown rice**

Place broth or water in a medium saucepan; add salt, if desired. Heat to boiling. Stir in rice and cover. Reduce heat to low and simmer for 40 minutes or until all the liquid has been absorbed. Fluff with a fork and serve. Makes 6 cups (twelve $\frac{1}{2}$-cup servings).

Note: To freeze single servings of brown rice, pack $\frac{1}{2}$ cup cooled cooked rice into small resealable freezer bags. Freeze up to 3 months. To serve, reheat for 2 to 3 minutes in the microwave oven.

Rice and Beans

$\frac{1}{2}$ **cup long grain brown rice, cooked**
$\frac{1}{2}$ **cup cooked beans (any kind)**

Combine rice and beans in a small saucepan. Cook until heated through, adding water if necessary. Serves 1.

Egg White Fried Rice

Toss 1 cup cooked long grain brown rice with scrambled egg whites. Heat and stir in a small skillet with $\frac{1}{2}$ cup reduced-sodium soy sauce and 2 teaspoons grated Parmesan cheese. Serves 2.

SIDES

Quinoa

2 cups water or low-fat chicken or vegetable broth
1 cup quinoa

Heat water or broth in a medium saucepan to boiling; stir in quinoa. Cover and reduce heat to low. Cover and simmer about 15 minutes or until quinoa is tender. Let stand for 5 minutes; fluff with a fork and serve. Serves 4.

Note: Quinoa can also be prepared in a rice cooker.

Baked Potato

Using a fork, poke several holes in a baking potato. Microwave for 7 to 8 minutes. Broil 1 to 2 minutes to make skins crunchy. Cut a slice from top of potato. Scoop out inside. Combine potato and 1 tablespoon Smart Balance® Buttery Spread or light sour cream. Spoon potato mixture back into potato shell, if desired. Serves 1.

SIDES

Lentils

1 tablespoon olive oil
1 medium onion, chopped
1 clove garlic, minced
1 cup dried lentils
1½ cups water or low-fat chicken or vegetable broth
½ teaspoon chopped fresh thyme or ½ teaspoon dried thyme, crushed

Heat a medium saucepan over medium-high heat for 2 minutes. Add olive oil and onions and saute until onions begin to soften. Add garlic and cook for 1 minute. Add lentils, water, and thyme and bring to a boil. Cover and reduce the heat to low. Simmer about 20 minutes or until lentils are tender. (Cooking time may vary.) Serves 4.

Other Grain Options:

Eddie's Organic® whole wheat pasta with soy
Whole Foods® soybean spaghetti
½ of a yam
Grilled eggplant
Corn on the cob
Artichoke dipped in hummus
La Tortilla Factory® Whole Wheat Tortillas for wraps
¼ cup All-Bran® for yogurt topping
Low-fat Triscuits® to serve with salads
Oroweat® Light Whole Wheat bread

SIDES

Asparagus Wrap-Ups

2 teaspoons light mayonnaise
1 teaspoon Dijon mustard
4 slices low-fat/low-salt ham
4 cooked asparagus spears

Mix mayonnaise and mustard together in a small bowl. Place a slice of ham on a plate; spread a thin layer of mustard mixture over ham. Wrap ham around an asparagus spear. Repeat with remaining ham, mustard mixture, and asparagus spears. Serves 1.

Not Your Mother's Onion Dip

1 tablespoon canola oil
1 large onion, halved and very thinly sliced
1 cup low-fat cottage cheese
½ cup fat-free plain yogurt (preferably Greek-style)
Freshly ground pepper
Cut-up veggies for dipping

Heat canola oil in a large skillet over medium heat. Add onion; reduce heat to low. Cook about 20 minutes or until golden brown, stirring occasionally. Remove from heat; cool. Place cottage cheese and yogurt in a food processor; blend until smooth. Add onion and pulse until blended but not pureed. Season to taste with pepper. Serve dip with cut-up veggies. Serves 2.

SNACKS

Parmesan Crisps with Smoked Turkey

1   **cup finely shredded Parmesan cheese**
    Freshly ground pepper
4   **ounces low-sodium smoked turkey breast, thinly sliced**

Heat a large nonstick skillet or griddle over medium-low heat. For each crisp, shape 2 tablespoons cheese to make a mound; drop it into the hot skillet. Repeat with remaining cheese for a total of 8 mounds, leaving 2 inches between each in the skillet. (Work in batches, if necessary.) Gently flatten mounds with the back of a spoon or spatula. Cook without disturbing them until they are crisp and golden, turning if necessary to cook evenly. (You may not need to turn them over, depending on how thick they are.) Carefully remove crisps from skillet; cool on waxed paper (crisps will become firm as they cool). Season to taste with pepper. Top with turkey. Serves 8.

Edamame Salad

1   **cup shelled edamame, cooked**
1   **cup grated carrot**
1   **scallion, chopped**
1   **tablespoon rice wine vinegar**
1   **tablespoon fresh lime juice**
1   **teaspoon canola oil**
2   **tablespoons chopped cilantro**

Combine edamame, carrot, and scallion in a bowl. Mix vinegar, lime juice, and canola oil and add to vegetables. Sprinkle with chopped cilantro. Serves 2.

SNACKS

Cucumber Boats

Create these fun grab-and-go snacks ahead of time. Start with a 6-inch piece of hothouse cucumber. Slice the cucumber in half lengthwise and use a teaspoon to scoop out the seeds. Use the hollow boats to make one of the delicious snacks on these two pages.

Caprese Gondolas

1 teaspoon prepared basil pesto
2 cucumber boats
1 small roma tomato, sliced into 4 rounds
1 small ball (1 ounce) water-pack fresh mozzarella cheese, sliced into 4 rounds

Spread a dollop of pesto in each of the cucumber boats. Place tomatoes and cheese inside each boat. Serves 2.

Mediterranean Yachts

4 tablespoons hummus
2 cucumber boats
1 bottled roasted red bell pepper, cut into strips

Spread 2 tablespoons of hummus in each cucumber boat. Top with roasted pepper strips. Serves 2.

Cottage Canoes

2   **cucumber boats**
½   **cup low-fat cottage cheese**
2   **tablespoons chopped walnuts**

Fill each cucumber boat with half of the cottage cheese. Top each with half of the nuts. Serves 2.

Submarines

3   **to 4 ounces sliced turkey breast**
2   **cucumber boats**
1   **stick low-fat string cheese, halved lengthwise**

Layer turkey in each cucumber boat. Top each boat with a piece of cheese. Serves 2.

Tuna Tubs

3   **to 4 ounces water-pack tuna, drained and flaked**
¼   **cup plain fat-free yogurt**
½   **teaspoon curry powder**
2   **cucumber boats**

Mix together tuna, yogurt, and curry powder in a small bowl. Spoon into cucumber boats. Serves 2.

SNACKS

More Snacks

✳ Stuff celery sticks with 1 to 1½ tablespoons soy nut butter, almond butter, or natural crunchy peanut butter.

✳ Spread bell pepper halves or quarters with 2 wedges of Laughing Cow® light cheese.

✳ Flake one 5-ounce pouch Starkist® tuna. If you like, season the tuna with chopped fresh dill, lemon juice, chopped scallion, and/or lemon pepper or combine tuna with a little light mayonnaise. Wrap tuna in lettuce leaves.

✳ Top 2 seaweed wraps with 2 ounces light cheese and 4 ounces turkey slices; roll up.

✳ Serve 2 hard-cooked egg whites, cauliflower florets, or celery sticks with 1 to 1½ tablespoons hummus.

✳ Serve 1 green apple with 1 string cheese.

✳ Serve 2 ounces turkey, beef, or salmon jerky with ½ or 1 medium cucumber, sliced.

✳ Serve 1 cup sugar snap peas with 1 ounce light Jarlsberg cheese.

✳ Stir together ¾ cup organic low-fat or fat-free plain yogurt and ½ cup fresh berries.

✳ Combine ½ cup fat-free cottage cheese with ½ cup berries, sliced kiwi, or cut-up cantaloupe.

✳ Serve 15 to 20 almonds with jicama slices or 8 to 10 almonds with a small pear.

✳ Serve ¾ cup cooked shelled edamame.

✳ Serve 1 to 2 tablespoons ricotta cheese, feta cheese, or hummus with celery sticks or bell pepper strips.

✳ Wrap 4 steamed asparagus spears with 4 ounces cooked sliced turkey.

✳ Serve 1 hard-cooked egg with steamed asparagus; drizzle with a little balsamic vinegar.

✳ Stir a little salsa into ½ cup low-fat cottage cheese.

✳ Serve 1 wedge cantaloupe with ½ cup cottage cheese.

✳ Wrap 2 to 3 ounces roasted turkey (spread turkey with mustard, if desired) around ¼ of a sliced peeled avocado.

✳ Sprinkle 1 cup plain low-fat or fat-free cottage cheese with ½ of an apple, chopped; ground cinnamon; and ground nutmeg.

✳ Serve ½ cup low-fat or fat-free cottage cheese with green beans.

SNACKS

Blue Berry Sunrise Shake

1 **cup water, plain soymilk, or fat-free milk**
1 **cup fresh or frozen boysenberries or ¾ cup blackberries or blueberries**
1 **scoop (2 tablespoons) vanilla or chocolate protein powder (whey, egg white, or soy)**

Combine water, berries, and protein powder in blender. Cover and blend until smooth. For a thicker shake, use less liquid. For an icier shake, add ice. Serves 1.

Red Berry Sunrise Shake

1 **cup water, plain soymilk, or fat-free milk**
1 **cup fresh or frozen raspberries or strawberries**
1 **scoop (2 tablespoons) vanilla or chocolate protein powder (whey, egg white, or soy)**

Combine water, berries, and protein powder in blender. Cover and blend until smooth. For a thicker shake, use less liquid. For an icier shake, add ice. Serves 1.

SHAKES

Mango Tango

1   cup water, plain soymilk, or fat-free milk
1   cup frozen mango or papaya chunks
1   scoop (2 tablespoons) vanilla protein powder (whey, egg white, or soy)
1   tablespoon wheat germ

Combine water, mango, protein powder, and wheat germ in a blender. Cover and blend until smooth. For a thicker shake, use less liquid. For an icier shake, add ice. Serves 1.

Tropical Chiller

1   cup water, plain soymilk or fat-free milk
½   cup drained canned pineapple tidbits (juice pack)
1   scoop (2 tablespoons) vanilla protein powder (whey, egg white, or soy)
⅛   teaspoon coconut or almond extract

Combine water, pineapple, protein powder, and coconut extract in a blender. Cover and blend until smooth. For a thicker shake, use less liquid. For an icier shake, add ice. Serves 1.

SHAKES

Choco-Monkey Protein Shake

1 cup water, plain soymilk, or fat-free milk
1 small banana or ½ of a medium banana, frozen if desired
1 scoop (2 tablespoons) chocolate protein powder (whey, egg white, or soy)
1 tablespoon ground flaxseed or flax oil

Combine water, banana, protein powder, and flaxseed in a blender. Cover and blend until smooth. For a thicker shake, use less liquid. For an icier shake, add ice. Serves 1.

Peanut Butter & Banana Shake

1 cup water, plain soymilk or fat-free milk
1 small banana or ½ of a medium banana, frozen if desired
1 scoop (2 tablespoons) vanilla or chocolate protein powder (whey, egg white, or soy)
1 tablespoon reduced-fat natural peanut butter

Combine water, banana, protein powder, and peanut butter in a blender. Cover and blend until smooth. For a thicker shake, use less liquid. For an icier shake, add ice. Serves 1.

Apple à la Mode Shake

1 cup water, plain soymilk, or fat-free milk
½ of an apple, chopped
1 scoop (2 tablespoons) vanilla protein powder (whey, egg white, or soy)
¼ teaspoon ground cinnamon

Combine water, apple, protein powder, and cinnamon in a blender. Cover and blend until smooth. For a thicker shake, use less liquid. For an icier shake, add ice. Serves 1.

SHAKES

Baked Apples

½ cup chopped walnuts
3 tablespoons roughly chopped dried cranberries
2 tablespoons packed brown sugar
½ teaspoon cinnamon
4 large firm baking apples, cored but not peeled
½ cup apple juice or apple cider
2 tablespoons maple syrup
Plain fat-free yogurt

Preheat the oven to 400°F. Stir together the nuts, dried cranberries, brown sugar, and cinnamon in a small bowl; set aside. Place the apples in a baking dish and spoon the nut mixture into the apples. Stir together apple juice and maple syrup; pour into the bottom of the baking dish.

Bake apples, uncovered, in the preheated oven for 25 to 35 minutes or until tender, basting occasionally with liquid in dish. Cool slightly before serving. Serve with yogurt. Serves 4.

DESSERTS

Granola-Topped Peaches

½   cup low-fat granola
1   egg white
¼   cup chopped almonds
4   ripe but firm peaches, halved and pitted
1   6-ounce container of vanilla (or plain) low-fat yogurt (optional)

Preheat oven to 350°F. Crush granola in a plastic bag. Transfer granola to a small bowl. Add egg white and almonds to granola; mix well. Arrange the peach halves, cut sides up, in a baking dish. Mound granola mixture on top of peach halves.

Bake in preheated oven about 45 minutes or until the topping is crisp and the peaches are tender. Serve with yogurt, if desired. Serves 4.

Grilled Pineapple

1   slice of fresh pineapple, ½ inch thick
½   cup plain nonfat yogurt, cottage cheese, or ricotta cheese (optional)

Preheat a grill pan over medium-high heat. Place the pineapple slice on the heated grill pan and cook on both sides until grill marks form and the pineapple is heated through. Transfer to a plate. Top with yogurt, if desired. Serves 1.

DESSERTS

Individual Ricotta Cheesecakes

6 ounces reduced-fat cream cheese (Neufchâtel), softened
¾ cup part-skim ricotta cheese
2 tablespoons honey
1 teaspoon grated lemon zest or 1 teaspoon grated fresh ginger
1 teaspoon vanilla extract
3 egg whites
Sliced strawberries or blueberries or all-fruit jam
Fresh mint leaves (optional)

Preheat oven to 350°F. Line 10 muffin cups with paper liners. Combine cream cheese, ricotta cheese, honey, lemon zest, and vanilla in a large bowl. Whisk together until well combined; set aside.

Place egg whites in a large mixing bowl. Beat with an electric mixer on medium speed until soft peaks form. Gently fold the egg whites into the cheese mixture. Divide evenly among the muffin cups.

Place muffin pan on the middle rack of the preheated oven. Bake for 15 to 18 minutes or until set. Remove from the oven. Cheesecakes will be puffed but will fall as they cool. When the cheesecakes have cooled, place in an airtight container and refrigerate for 2 hours or overnight. Just before serving, top with berries or jam (½ teaspoon jam per cheesecake). Garnish with mint, if desired. Makes 10 cheesecakes.

Breakfast Ricotta Cheesecakes: Prepare cheesecakes as above, except omit the honey, lemon zest, and vanilla. Add 2 tablespoons grated Parmesan cheese to cream cheese mixture. Before serving, top cheesecakes with chopped tomato and chopped fresh basil.

DESSERTS

Banana-Nut Pops

4 wooden sticks or short bamboo skewers
2 firm ripe bananas, peeled and halved crosswise
4 12-inch squares aluminum foil
1 ounce 70 percent dark chocolate, finely grated
1 tablespoon creamy peanut butter

Insert a wooden stick into each banana half. Place each on a square of foil. Place the chocolate on a plate. Heat the peanut butter in a small dish in the microwave oven until barely warm but spreadable. Coat each banana half with a thin layer of peanut butter; roll in the chocolate. Wrap each banana tightly in foil. Freeze at least 2 hours or up to 2 weeks. Serves 4.

Frozen Grapes

1 small bunch seedless red grapes (about ½ cup)

Rinse the grapes very well and let dry on a towel. Remove the grapes from the stems and place in a resealable freezer bag. Freeze for at least 2 hours or up to 1 week. Serves 1 (½ cup).

DESSERTS

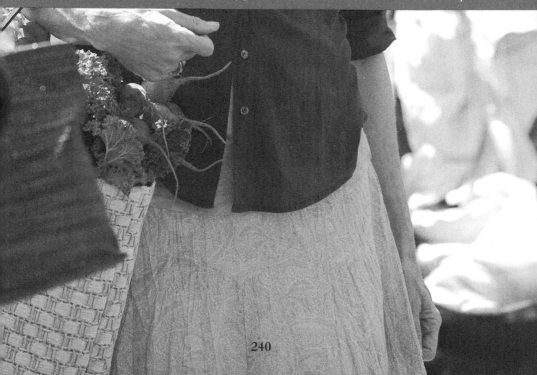

KATHY'S CALIFORNIA RESTAURANT FAVORITES

California is a chef's paradise since there's always a variety of fresh produce available. Here some of my favorite restaurants share their recipes.

A Votre Santé, *Brentwood, California*

Tex-Mex Scramble

4 tablespoons olive oil, divided
4 egg whites
4 ounces salmon, cut into 4 strips
2 tablespoons Cajun Seasoning (recipe follows) or purchased Cajun seasoning
2 tablespoons minced red onion
2 tablespoons roasted red bell pepper*
½ jalapeño chile pepper, seeded and chopped
1 clove garlic, minced
4 corn tortillas
2 tablespoons canned tomato sauce
2 tablespoons water
2 tablespoons shredded cheddar cheese or soy cheese
1 tablespoon chopped fresh cilantro
1 tablespoon chopped scallion
   Sea salt and ground pepper

Heat 1 tablespoon of the oil in a nonstick skillet. Cook and stir egg whites in skillet until scrambled; set aside. Coat salmon with Cajun Seasoning. Heat 1 tablespoon of the remaining oil in same skillet; cook fish until blackened; set aside. Wipe skillet clean. Cook red onion, roasted pepper, jalapeño pepper, and garlic in remaining 2 tablespoons oil until softened.

Chop 3 of the tortillas. Add chopped tortillas, tomato sauce, and water to skillet; cook until tortillas are soft. Add the egg whites, the salmon, the cheese, cilantro, and scallion; cook and stir until heated through. Season with salt and ground pepper. Serve on the remaining tortilla and, if desired, with salsa or guacamole, black or pinto beans, and tortilla chips.

Cajun Seasoning: Combine 4 tablespoons paprika, 2 tablespoons mild chili powder, 1 teaspoon ground cumin, 1 teaspoon Italian seasoning, ½ teaspoon sea salt, and ¼ teaspoon black pepper. Makes about ½ cup.

*Note: To roast bell pepper, rub pepper with olive oil. Roast over a medium flame for 15 minutes or until charred. Place pepper in a paper bag for 20 minutes. Remove skin. Cut pepper in half; remove ribs and seeds. Chop.

FAVORITES

Mogan's Café *Pacific Palisades, California*

Kathy's Favorite Omelet

    Nonstick olive oil cooking spray
¼ **cup lightly packed spinach**
1 **medium tomato, sliced**
¼ **of a peeled avocado, sliced**
3 **egg whites**
    Sea salt and ground pepper

Coat a nonstick skillet with cooking spray. Heat the skillet over medium heat. Add spinach to skillet; cook over medium heat until wilted. Add tomato and avocado. Reduce heat to low.

Beat the egg whites in a small bowl until combined; whisk 30 seconds more. Pour the egg whites into the skillet over vegetables. Stir with a rubber spatula, lifting cooked eggs to allow liquid egg to flow underneath. Continue until egg whites are almost set. Slide omelet to a plate; fold in half. Season to taste with sea salt and pepper. Serves 1.

FAVORITES

Wilshire Restaurant *Santa Monica, California*

Gazpacho Soup

6   medium heirloom (Brandywine) tomatoes or other vine-ripened
    tomatoes (2 pounds)
8   ounces cucumber, peeled, seeded, and chopped
1   medium fennel bulb, trimmed and chopped
½   of a red bell pepper, chopped
¼   cup chopped fresh Italian (flat-leaf) parsley
2   cups tomato juice
1   cup extra virgin olive oil
3   tablespoons sherry vinegar
3   tablespoons sugar (or to taste)
1   small clove garlic, minced
¼   teaspoon cayenne pepper
1   teaspoon fine sea salt
½   teaspoon freshly ground black pepper
    Gazpacho Garnish (recipe follows)
12 large cooked shrimp, peeled, deveined, and chilled
6   sprigs fresh cilantro
6   lime wedges

Coarsely chop tomatoes. Combine tomatoes, cucumber, fennel, bell pepper, parsley, tomato juice, oil, vinegar, sugar, and garlic in a bowl. Cover; chill for 1 hour.

Process tomato mixture, in batches, in a food processor until almost pureed but still coarse in texture. Return all of the mixture to the bowl. Stir in cayenne pepper, sea salt, and ground pepper. Cover and chill for at least 1 hour.

To serve, ladle 1½ cups of the soup into chilled shallow soup bowls. Spoon ¼ cup Gazpacho Garnish onto center of each serving. Top with shrimp and cilantro sprigs. Garnish with lime wedges. Serves 6.

Gazpacho Garnish: Combine 2 tablespoons chopped red bell pepper, 2 tablespoons chopped yellow bell pepper, 2 tablespoons chopped red onion, ½ cup coarsely chopped red and yellow cherry tomatoes, ½ cup chopped cilantro leaves, and ¼ cup lime juice in a medium bowl. Season to taste with sea salt and freshly ground black pepper.

Rosti *Santa Monica, California*

Turkey Chopped Salad

8 **cups mixed baby greens**
1 **pound roma tomatoes, chopped**
8 **ounces Homemade Roast Turkey Breast (recipe follows) or leftover turkey,**
   chopped (about 1½ cups)
1 **sprig fresh basil, chopped**
1 **tablespoon extra virgin olive oil**
½ **cup Balsamic Dressing (recipe follows)**
   Salt and ground pepper

Combine baby greens, tomatoes, turkey, basil, and olive oil in a large bowl. Drizzle with Balsamic Dressing; toss to coat. Season to taste with salt and pepper. Serves 2.

Homemade Roast Turkey Breast: Preheat oven to 400°F. Place a 3- to 4-pound turkey breast in a shallow roasting pan. Rub turkey breast with 2 tablespoons olive oil; 1 sprig sage, chopped; 1 sprig rosemary, chopped; 2 cloves garlic, crushed; dash salt; and dash ground pepper. Insert a meat thermometer into the turkey breast. Add ½ cup vegetable broth to pan. Roast about 1½ hours or until thermometer registers 165°F, basting turkey with pan juices every 30 minutes. Makes about 2 pounds cooked turkey.

Balsamic Dressing: Whisk together ½ cup extra virgin olive oil, ¼ cup balsamic vinegar, 2 tablespoons red wine, and 1 tablespoon Dijon mustard in a small bowl. Season to taste with salt and ground pepper. Makes 1 cup.

Michael's *Santa Monica, California*

Grilled Chicken and Goat Cheese Salad

6   chicken breast halves, boned with skin and wing bones attached
1   log (12 ounces) fresh creamy white California goat cheese, cut into
    ¼-inch medallions
    Salt and freshly ground pepper
3   red bell peppers, cut into ¾- to 1-inch strips
3   yellow bell peppers, cut into ¾- to 1-inch strips
1   large or 2 medium Maui, Walla Walla, Vidalia, or sweet red onions, cut into
    ⅜-inch slices
2   tablespoons extra virgin olive oil
3   heads mâche, torn into bite-size pieces
2   bunches arugula, torn into bite-size pieces
2   heads baby red leaf lettuce, torn into bite-size pieces
1   head radicchio, separated into leaves
1   cup tomato concassé or chopped tomatoes
1   cup balsamic vinaigrette
1   cup jalapeño-cilantro-lime salsa
1   bunch fresh chives, finely chopped

Preheat grill or broiler. With your finger, gently make a pocket between the skin and meat of each chicken breast. Insert the goat cheese medallions into the pockets, overlapping cheese as necessary. Sprinkle chicken with salt and ground pepper. Brush bell peppers and onion with olive oil. Sprinkle with salt and ground pepper; set aside.

Place chicken on grill rack, skin sides up, over medium heat. Grill for 3 to 5 minutes or until browned. Turn chicken over; grill for 5 to 7 minutes more. Add bell peppers and onion to grill. Grill about 1 minute or until chicken is done and vegetables are heated through and slightly charred, turning once. (Or broil chicken and vegetables 4 to 5 inches from heat.)

Arrange mâche, arugula, lettuce, and radicchio on 6 plates. Cut each chicken breast into 4 slices and place on the plates. Add tomato concassé, grilled peppers, and onions to plates. Drizzle vinaigrette over vegetables. Spoon salsa over chicken. Sprinkle with chives. Serves 6.

FAVORITES

Wilshire Restaurant *Santa Monica, California*

Niçoise Salad with Seared Tuna

2 pounds sushi grade ahi tuna, cut into 4×2×2-inch pieces
   Sea salt and freshly ground pepper
1 tablespoon extra virgin olive oil
1 pound French haricots verts or tiny green beans, trimmed
1 pound baby purple artichokes, trimmed
2 pounds tiny new potatoes
1 pound mixed baby greens
1 red bell pepper, cut into ¼-inch strips
1 yellow bell pepper, cut into ¼-inch strips
   Niçoise Vinaigrette (recipe follows)
4 ounces red and/or yellow cherry tomatoes
20 white anchovy fillets in oil, drained and patted dry
5 hard-cooked eggs, quartered lengthwise
1 cup Niçoise olives

Sprinkle tuna with sea salt and freshly ground black pepper. Heat olive oil in a large skillet over medium-high heat. Add tuna; sear on all sides until done but rare. Let stand a few minutes; cut into ¼-inch slices. Set aside.

Bring 6 cups water to boiling in large saucepan. Add half of the haricots verts; cook just until tender, 3 to 4 minutes. Remove beans and plunge into ice water to cool. Repeat with remaining beans and the artichokes. Set beans and artichokes aside. Add potatoes to boiling water; cook for 10 to 12 minutes, Drain; plunge in ice water to cool. When cool, peel potatoes.

For salad, toss together greens, beans, artichokes, and red and yellow bell pepper strips in a large bowl. Drizzle with some of the Niçoise Vinaigrette; toss to coat. Season with salt and ground pepper. Arrange greens mixture in center of a serving platter. Arrange tuna, potatoes, cherry tomatoes, anchovies, and eggs on top. Sprinkle with olives. Drizzle with remaining vinaigrette. Garnish with parsley and chervil, if desired. Serves 8 to 10.

Niçoise Vinaigrette: Whisk together 3 tablespoons sherry vinegar, 3 tablespoons red wine vinegar, and 1 tablespoon Dijon mustard in a small bowl. Add 1 cup extra virgin olive oil in a thin stream, whisking to emulsify. Season with lemon juice, sea salt, and freshly ground black pepper.

Border Grill *Santa Monica, California*

Halibut Veracruzana

- 3 tablespoons extra virgin olive oil
- 1½ pounds boneless, skinless Pacific halibut fillets, cut into 4 portions
  Salt and freshly ground pepper
- 1 small onion, thinly sliced
- 2 cloves garlic, minced
- 2 to 3 jalapeño chile peppers, sliced and seeded
- 1 lime, cut into 8 wedges
- 1 medium tomato, cut into wedges and seeded
- ½ cup Spanish green olives (picholines), sliced
- ½ of a bunch fresh oregano, roughly chopped
- ½ cup dry white wine
- ¾ cup fish stock or clam juice

Heat a very large skillet or two medium saute pans over medium-high heat for 1 minute; add olive oil. Sprinkle fish with salt and ground pepper. Sear fish in hot oil in pan(s) until golden on both sides, turning once. Remove fish to a rack placed over a plate to catch juices.

Add onion to pan(s); cook and stir over medium-high heat for 2 minutes. Add garlic, chile peppers, lime wedges, tomato, olives, and oregano. Cook and stir for 1 minute more. Add white wine; bring to boiling. Cook until wine is reduced by half. Add fish stock and bring to a boil. Return fish along with juices to pan(s). Cook, covered, 1 to 3 minutes or until fish begins to flake. Season broth with salt and ground pepper to taste. Transfer fillets to 4 soup bowls. Spoon broth over fish; top with vegetables. Serves 4.

FAVORITES

Melisse Restaurant *Santa Monica, California*

Dover Sole "Roasted on the Bone"

2 **14-ounce whole Dover sole, skins removed and bones trimmed**
   All-purpose flour
1 **tablespoon olive oil**
4 **tablespoons unsalted butter**
¼ **cup water**
2 **tablespoons lemon juice**
1 **tablespoon chopped fresh parsley**
1 **tablespoon capers**
1 **tablespoon chopped tomato**

Preheat oven to 400°F. Sprinkle fish with salt and black pepper. Dredge fish
in flour. Heat oil and 1 tablespoon of the butter in ovenproof skillet. Add fish;
cook in hot oil about 5 minutes or until golden on one side. Add 1 tablespoon
of the remaining butter. Turn the fish over and cook for 2 minutes. Place in
the oven about 5 minutes or until fish flakes easily with a fork. Baste fish with
butter in pan. Remove fish from pan. Remove side fins. Separate top fillets and
slide them off the bone. Pull up and remove backbones. Reassemble the fish.

For sauce, heat remaining 2 tablespoons butter in small saute pan over high
heat just until brown. Add the water and lemon juice. Reduce heat to low. Stir
in the parsley, capers, and tomato. Season to taste with salt and ground pepper
and remove from heat. Arrange fish, Creamed Spinach, and Cooked Spinach
(recipes follow) on two dinner plates. Spoon sauce over fish. Serves 2.

Creamed Spinach: Heat 1 teaspoon olive oil and 1 teaspoon unsalted butter
in a large saucepan over medium heat. Add 1 clove garlic, minced, and
1 teaspoon finely chopped shallots. Cook 1 minute (do not brown). Add 2 cups
firmly packed spinach; cook just until wilted. Add 1 tablespoon heavy cream;
cook until desired consistency. Season to taste with salt and pepper. Transfer
to a blender; blend until smooth.

Cooked Spinach: Cook 3 cups firmly packed spinach in boiling salted water
for 5 minutes. Remove and place in ice water. Drain well, squeezing excess
water from spinach.

JiRaffe, *Santa Monica, California*

Roasted Chicken with Garden Ragoût

4 8-ounce chicken breast halves with winglet attached
2 tablespoons olive oil
½ cup butter
 Garden Ragoût (recipe follows)
1 teaspoon chopped fresh thyme
½ cup Roasted Chicken Jus (recipe follows)

Preheat oven to 500°F. Sprinkle chicken with salt and ground pepper. Heat oil in large ovenproof skillet. Add chicken, skin sides down. Reduce heat; cook for 3 minutes. Place skillet in oven; bake 9 to 11 minutes or until done. For emulsified butter, bring ⅓ cup water and 1 teaspoon of the butter to boiling in saucepan. Whisk in remaining butter; bring to boiling. Season with salt and pepper. Heat Garden Ragoût in another saucepan. Add thyme and emulsified butter; keep warm. Remove chicken from oven; place, skin sides up on plate. Drain fat from skillet; add Roasted Chicken Jus to skillet; bring to boiling. Season to taste. Serve chicken with ragoût and sauce. Serves 4.

Garden Ragoût: In a saute pan cook 12 peeled pearl onions with ¼ cup water, 2 tablespoons butter, and 1 tablespoon sugar over medium heat until liquid has evaporated and onions are glazed. Remove from pan. In same pan cook 12 peeled garlic cloves with 3 tablespoons olive oil until golden. Mix together onions, garlic, ½ cup cooked white corn kernels, ½ cup cooked peas, and ½ cup diced cooked potatoes.

Roasted Chicken Jus: Preheat oven to 350°F. In a heavy roasting pan brown 1 to 2 pounds chicken carcasses or bones (chopped into 2-inch pieces) in 1 teaspoon olive oil. Roast in oven 15 minutes, stirring halfway through. Add ⅓ cup coarsely chopped carrot, ¼ cup coarsely chopped onion, and 2 cloves crushed unpeeled garlic. Roast 15 minutes or until well caramelized. Return pan to stovetop; add ½ cup white wine and 1 sprig fresh thyme. Cook over medium heat, stirring and scraping bottom and sides of pan, until wine has almost completely evaporated. Add 2 cups chicken stock and simmer, stirring occasionally, until it has reduced to about 1 cup liquid. Press mixture through a strainer lined with a double thickness of cheesecloth. Discard solids.

FAVORITES

DIET INDEX

RECIPE INDEX

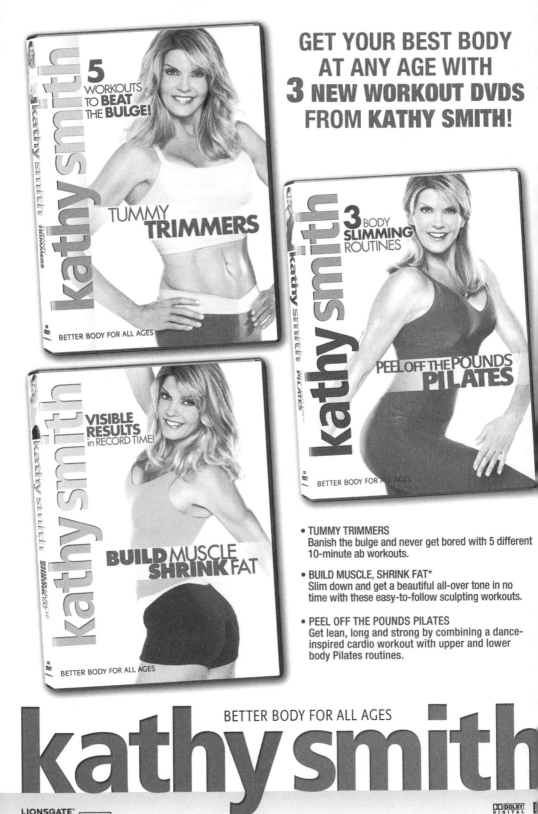